I0707896

Carb Cycling for Weight Loss for Women Over 50

A Complete Cookbook for Beginners to Lose Weight, Build Power, and Boost Energy with Easy-to-Follow Exercise Plan and Delicious Recipes + Bonus: 21 Day Meal Plan + Audiobook + Video Course

Dr. Valerie Kennedy

Copyright © 2024 by Dr. Valerie Kennedy

All rights reserved. No part of this publication may be reproduced, distributed, or transmitted in any form or by any means, including photocopying, recording, or other electronic or mechanical methods, without the prior written permission of the publisher, except in the case of brief quotations embodied in critical reviews and certain other noncommercial uses permitted by copyright law. For permission requests, write to the publisher at the address below.

Disclaimer!

The information provided in this [book/article/website/etc.] is for general informational purposes only. While every effort has been made to provide accurate and up-to-date information, Dr. Valerie Kennedy makes no representations or warranties of any kind, express or implied, about the completeness, accuracy, reliability, suitability, or availability of the information contained herein for any purpose. Any reliance you place on such information is therefore strictly at your own risk.

Bonus

21-Day Meal Plan

Day 1

Breakfast: Overnight Chia Seed Pudding with Berries
Lunch: Grilled Chicken and Veggie Bowl with Quinoa
Dinner: Whole Grain Veggie Lasagna with Ground Turkey
Snack 1: Greek Yogurt with Mixed Berries and Nuts
Snack 2: Apple Slices with Almond Butter

Day 2

Breakfast: Spinach and Feta Egg Muffins
Lunch: Turkey and Veggie Stuffed Peppers
Dinner: Grilled Salmon with Roasted Veggies
Snack 1: Whole Grain Crackers with Hummus and Veggies
Snack 2: Banana and Peanut Butter Roll-Ups

Day 3

Breakfast: Avocado Toast with Smoked Salmon
Lunch: Whole Grain Pasta Salad with Veggies and Feta
Dinner: Chicken and Veggie Stir-Fry with Brown Rice
Snack 1: Mixed Berry and Greek Yogurt Parfait
Snack 2: Turkey and Cheese Roll-Ups with Spinach

Day 4

Breakfast: Protein Pancakes with Almond Butter
Lunch: Shrimp and Veggie Skewers with Quinoa
Dinner: Turkey and Veggie Chili with Whole Grain Bread
Snack 1: High-Protein Oatmeal with Mixed Berries
Snack 2: Veggie and Hummus Pita Pocket

Day 5

Breakfast: Sweet Potato and Kale Hash
Lunch: Whole Grain Veggie Pizza with Mozzarella
Dinner: Grilled Chicken and Veggie Skewers with Brown Rice
Snack 1: Mixed Berry and Spinach Smoothie
Snack 2: Whole Grain Energy Bites with Nuts and Seeds

Day 6

Breakfast: Whole Grain Waffles with Fresh Fruit
Lunch: Chicken and Veggie Fried Rice
Dinner: Turkey and Veggie Meatloaf with Roasted Sweet Potatoes
Snack 1: Cottage Cheese and Fruit Plate
Snack 2: Peanut Butter and Banana Smoothie

Day 7

Breakfast: Low-Carb Breakfast Burritos with Egg and Cheese
Lunch: Grilled Veggie and Hummus Pita Pocket
Dinner: Whole Grain Pasta with Chicken and Veggies
Snack 1: Whole Grain Crackers with Cheese and Turkey
Snack 2: Greek Yogurt and Granola with Mixed Berries

Day 8

Breakfast: Veggie-Packed Omelet
Lunch: Turkey and Cheese Lettuce Wraps
Dinner: Shrimp and Veggie Fried Rice
Snack 1: High-Protein Smoothie Bowl
Snack 2: Whole Grain Blueberry Muffins

Day 9

Breakfast: High-Protein Oatmeal with Mixed Berries
Lunch: Whole Grain Veggie Pizza with Mozzarella
Dinner: Grilled Chicken and Veggie Skewers with Quinoa
Snack 1: Turkey and Cheese Roll-Ups with Spinach

Snack 2: Mixed Berry and Spinach Smoothie

Day 10

Breakfast: Greek Yogurt Parfait with Nuts and Seeds
Lunch: Whole Grain Pasta Salad with Veggies and Feta
Dinner: Turkey and Veggie Shepherd's Pie with Sweet
Potato Topping
Snack 1: Whole Grain Toast with Avocado and Egg
Snack 2: Whole Grain Energy Bites with Nuts and Seeds

Day 11

Breakfast: Whole Grain French Toast with Fresh Fruit
Lunch: Chicken and Veggie Soup with Whole Grain
Crackers
Dinner: Grilled Salmon and Veggie Skewers with Brown
Rice
Snack 1: Veggie and Hummus Sandwich on Whole
Grain Bread
Snack 2: Banana and Peanut Butter Roll-Ups

Day 12

Breakfast: Low-Carb Breakfast Casserole with Veggies
and Cheese
Lunch: Whole Grain Veggie Lasagna with Ground
Turkey
Dinner: Whole Grain Pasta with Shrimp and Veggies
Snack 1: Greek Yogurt and Granola with Mixed Berries
Snack 2: Whole Grain Crackers with Hummus and
Veggies

Day 13

Breakfast: Egg and Veggie Breakfast Sandwich
Lunch: Turkey and Veggie Stuffed Acorn Squash
Dinner: Chicken and Veggie Fried Rice
Snack 1: High-Protein Smoothie Bowl
Snack 2: Cottage Cheese and Fruit Plate

Day 14

Breakfast: Quinoa Breakfast Bowl with Nuts and Seeds

Lunch: Grilled Chicken and Veggie Bowl with Quinoa
Dinner: Whole Grain Veggie Pizza with Mozzarella
Snack 1: Mixed Berry and Spinach Smoothie
Snack 2: Whole Grain Energy Bites with Nuts and Seeds

Day 15

Breakfast: High-Protein Oatmeal with Mixed Berries
Lunch: Whole Grain Pasta Salad with Veggies and Feta
Dinner: Turkey and Veggie Chili with Whole Grain
Bread
Snack 1: Whole Grain Crackers with Cheese and Turkey
Snack 2: Peanut Butter and Banana Smoothie

Day 16

Breakfast: Whole Grain Waffles with Fresh Fruit
Lunch: Grilled Veggie and Hummus Pita Pocket
Dinner: Chicken and Veggie Stir-Fry with Brown Rice
Snack 1: Greek Yogurt and Granola with Mixed Berries
Snack 2: Veggie and Hummus Sandwich on Whole
Grain Bread

Day 17

Breakfast: Veggie-Packed Omelet
Lunch: Whole Grain Veggie Lasagna with Ground
Turkey
Dinner: Grilled Chicken and Veggie Skewers with
Brown Rice
Snack 1: High-Protein Smoothie Bowl
Snack 2: Whole Grain Blueberry Muffins

Day 18

Breakfast: Low-Carb Breakfast Burritos with Egg and
Cheese
Lunch: Turkey and Veggie Stuffed Peppers
Dinner: Shrimp and Veggie Fried Rice
Snack 1: Whole Grain Crackers with Hummus and
Veggies
Snack 2: Banana and Peanut Butter Roll-Ups

Day 19

Breakfast: Greek Yogurt Parfait with Nuts and Seeds
Lunch: Whole Grain Pasta with Chicken and Veggies
Dinner: Turkey and Veggie Meatloaf with Roasted Sweet Potatoes
Snack 1: Cottage Cheese and Fruit Plate
Snack 2: Mixed Berry and Spinach Smoothie

Day 20

Breakfast: Whole Grain French Toast with Fresh Fruit
Lunch: Chicken and Veggie Soup with Whole Grain Crackers

Dinner: Grilled Salmon and Veggie Skewers with Brown Rice
Snack 1: Turkey and Cheese Roll-Ups with Spinach
Snack 2: Whole Grain Energy Bites with Nuts and Seeds

Day 21

Breakfast: Egg and Veggie Breakfast Sandwich
Lunch: Whole Grain Veggie Lasagna with Ground Turkey
Dinner: Whole Grain Pasta with Shrimp and Veggies
Snack 1: Greek Yogurt and Granola with Mixed Berries
Snack 2: Whole Grain Crackers with Cheese and Turkey

Here is one of the biggest bonuses I promised you…

A full Audiobook on the Carb cycling diet

To get access to it, kindly type in this link on your browser:
http://tinyurl.com/mxs3tns8

OR

Scan the below QR code to gain access.

About The Author

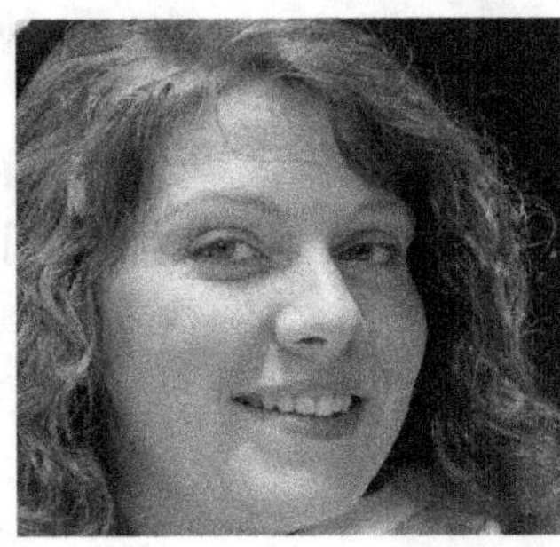 Renowned culinary expert and Culinary Institute of America alumna Dr. Valerie Kennedy is well recognized for her creative approach to food and in-depth knowledge of the many nutritional components that are included in every dish. For almost two decades, Dr. Kennedy has been a fixture in Michelin-starred restaurants' kitchens, showcasing his ability to blend traditional methods with contemporary, worldwide flare.

As an author, she celebrates the variety of cultures in her recipes while highlighting the link between our general health and what we eat. Dr. Kennedy's viewpoint on food is distinct since he considers cooking to be an artistic endeavor that feeds the body and the spirit, rather than merely a practical skill.

Connect with Dr. Valerie Kennedy:
Email: ***drvaleriekennedy@gmail.com***

Table Of Content

Introduction

A lady in her fifties—that's me—began her journey for a healthy living once upon a time, in a place full of contradicting advice and never-ending diets. I had no idea that this adventure would introduce me to a wealth of information and a group of passionate carb-cyclists.

I'm Valerie, and I'm here to tell you my tale. It's a story of learning via trial and error about the effectiveness of carb cycling and how it enhanced my energy, helped me gain strength, and helped me lose weight. To assist you on your own carb cycling journey, I've also included an audiobook, video course, and 21-day food plan as an extra bonus.

We are all too aware of the issue of weight gain at the start of my journey. I discovered that, as a woman over 50, my energy levels had decreased and my metabolism had slowed down. I was confused by the abundance of diets and contradicting advice, but I knew I had to change.

I experimented with a few other diets, but none of them gave me the desired effects or were not too restrictive. That's how I learned about carb cycling, a versatile and successful weight-loss strategy that alternates between days with high and low carbs.

I wasn't sure at first. How may consuming more carbohydrates aid in my weight loss efforts? However, when I learned more about the science behind carb cycling, I discovered that it was a well studied and reliable approach. It keeps metabolism from slowing down, helps control insulin levels, and even helps women over 50 produce more hormones.

I made the decision to try it. I began by making a meal plan and included simple-to-find components like healthy fats, lean meats, and whole grains. I was astounded by the range of delectable foods I could come up with using this method. In addition, I noticed that I had more energy and felt better about my physical appearance.

However, my adventure didn't stop there. I found that I wasn't the only one pursuing a healthy lifestyle as I persisted in adhering to the carb cycling regimen. I got to know others who were having comparable results with carb cycling. We exchanged recipes, told one other our experiences, and even formed a support group to keep each other motivated.

I realized I had to impart my newfound knowledge to others as I kept becoming stronger, losing weight, and having more energy. This is why I created the "Carb Cycling for Weight Loss for Women Over 50" program.

All the information you need to start your own carb cycling adventure is included within this book. This book is your one-stop resource for empowerment and weight reduction, with everything from simple-to-follow food planning and recipes to an exercise regimen created especially for women over 50.

And what's great about it? Not only myself have benefited from carb cycling. This strategy has worked well for my buddies and other carb cyclers. They've gained strength, shed pounds, and developed a renewed sense of self by adhering to the guidelines presented in this book.

What are you waiting for then? Come along on this journey with me as we explore the power of this adaptable and successful weight reduction strategy via carb cycling. You'll have all the resources and encouragement you need to reach your objectives and lead the greatest possible life when "Carb Cycling for Weight Loss for Women Over 50" is on your side.

Recall that there is a solution waiting for you on the other side of the page for your health and weight reduction problems. Obtain a copy of this fantastic book right now to get started on the path to a happier, healthier version of yourself.

Chapter 1: Understanding Carb Cycling

What is carb cycling

Serious bodybuilders and athletes who wish to lose body fat, gain muscle, or store more carbohydrates for long-distance exercises like marathons utilize an extremely rigid diet called carb cycling. Despite the fact that water makes up a large portion of the weight loss, it's growing in popularity among those looking to lose weight quickly.

Carbs are necessary for your body to function properly. Its energy comes from lipids, proteins, and carbohydrates and is expressed in calories. However, one gram of fat has nine calories, compared to only four from carbohydrates or proteins. Generally speaking, experts advise consuming 50% to 55% of your daily calories from carbohydrates, 10% to 15% from proteins, and less than 30% from fats.

Carbs come in several healthful varieties. Dairy products and plant-based meals such as grains, beans, fruits, and vegetables naturally contain them. Additionally, they are added as starches or sugars to processed meals.

Your body requires glucose, which is produced during the breakdown of carbohydrates, as fuel. You may have less cravings for carbohydrates and have more energy if you stop depending on them to power your body.

Going back and forth between high-carb and low-carb days is known as carb cycling. Some days may even be "no-carb."

Typically, you would eat a high-carb day if you intended to engage in vigorous exercise. You may need to consume 2 to 2.5 grams of carbohydrates for every pound of body weight on such days since your body requires more fuel.

On days when you're not as active, you consume less carbohydrates. You may have meals on low-carb days.for every pound of body weight, 5 grams of carbohydrates. A "no-carb" day is one in which you consume less than 30 grams of carbohydrates throughout the day.

Another approach is to stick to a three-day diet where you only consume 100–125 grams of carbohydrates every day. Next, on days when you are more active, you consume a lot of carbohydrates (175-275 grams) for two days.

How Carb Cycling Works

When you consume carbohydrate-containing meals and your blood sugar rises, your pancreas produces more insulin, a hormone that transports glucose into cells. There, the glucose is either stored for later use, transformed into fat, or converted into energy.

Your pancreas sends signals to your cells to release glucagon, which is stored glucose, when the cells take in blood sugar. This oscillation ensures that your body is getting the proper quantity of sugar.

But eating a diet high in carbohydrates might cause your body to produce too much insulin. This may result in weight gain and an increased risk of heart disease and type 2 diabetes.

Your body may be able to burn fat rather than carbohydrates and muscle tissue if you take brief pauses to cycle through carbohydrates. However, keep in mind that high-carb days may cause weight gain if you aren't exercising often or engaging in hard training during carb cycling.

Although the long-term consequences of carb cycling are not well studied, it is often safe to do so for brief periods of time. To regulate your blood pressure, blood sugar, and cholesterol, make sure your diet is healthy overall.

Benefits of carb cycling

Why would someone choose for a carb cycle as opposed to a traditional diet? Among the benefits of a carb cycling diet are:

1. Boosting weight loss or lowering body fat percentage; preserving muscle mass and preventing muscle wasting; assisting muscle recovery after workouts; preventing a dip in your metabolic rate by increasing leptin levels; one study found that a three-day plan that overfed on carbohydrates increased leptin and 24-hour energy expenditure, but a three-day plan that overfed on fat did not.
2. Letting you stick to your diet and continue eating your favorite foods; providing you with more energy; averting acute hunger or exhaustion; and assisting in the prevention of hormone imbalances

Here are a few additional details about the primary advantages of a carb cycling diet:

1. Helps Construct and Maintain Mass of Lean Muscle

Muscle tissue is really broken down by strength training and other resistance exercise methods, but it then grows back stronger. Again, your body needs part of its main fuel source—carbs—to maintain and repair muscle tissue, which is an energy-intensive operation. The term "post-workout anabolic window" refers to this period.

After consuming more carbohydrates, insulin controls the entrance of amino acids and glucose into muscle cells, which has significant anabolic benefits. A 2013 research that was published in the Journal of the International Society of Sports Nutrition revealed that carbohydrates make you feel more energized again and provide your muscles glucose to repair or glycogen to store for later. However, when dietary carbohydrates are limited, ketones may also function as a fuel source, which may be advantageous for some athletes. This is why many find that cycling works well for them.

"How many calories a day should I consume?" Following resistance training, you run the risk of "starving" your muscles of the nutrition they need to come back stronger and larger if you don't eat enough calories and carbs. This is why a lot of individuals who are serious about gaining muscle opt to have higher carb days after challenging exercises. Long-term improvements in physical performance may also result from consuming at least modest quantities of carbohydrates, according to some research.

Just cutting calories and increasing your exercise might have a negative impact on your metabolism and possibly have the opposite effect of what you want, making you feel weaker, more exhausted, and less able to eat without gaining weight. If you can schedule your higher and lower carbohydrate consumption days around your exercises, you can reduce your body fat percentage without compromising your muscle mass. Furthermore, bear in mind that maintaining your maximum muscle mass is essential for maintaining a healthy rate of calorie expenditure throughout old life.

2. Could Aid in Preventing a Decline in Your Metabolic Rate

In one research, the resting metabolic rate of 74 people who followed a "calorie shifting diet" (in which carbohydrates were also raised and reduced) for six weeks tended to stay stable. Additionally, they saw decreases in triacylglycerol, total cholesterol, and plasma glucose. Those following the calorie shifting plan reported feeling less hungry and more satisfied than those following the "classic calorie restriction diet."

3. Promotes Sustaining a Healthy Weight

Does carb cycling help people lose weight? It very definitely can be. A carb cycling diet's ability to maintain and even accelerate weight reduction while maintaining and even increasing lean muscle mass is one of its main advantages. This is the gold standard when it comes to changing body composition since it maintains your metabolism functioning at its peak and makes it easier for you to maintain your weight over the long term.

A "carb deficit," or consuming less carbohydrates than your body requires, promotes weight reduction because it causes your body to start burning fat that has been stored as fuel. Many individuals find that cutting their carbohydrates very low and adhering to diets like the Atkins or ketogenic diets helps them achieve a healthy weight and improve specific health concerns. However, for others, the hormonal fluctuations make it hard to maintain and, when followed over time, might actually slow down the metabolism.

One strategy to avoid gaining weight again and losing motivation is to carb cycle. It may also help you lose weight over the long run by providing you with energy and rapid results.

4. Inspires You to Consume More Plant-Based Foods

The majority of plant meals include carbohydrates as their main macronutrient, however the precise amount varies depending on the kind. On days with a greater carbohydrate content, whole foods like fruit, lentils and beans, sweet potatoes and other root vegetables, are often recommended.

Many of the world's healthiest foods, such leafy greens, cruciferous vegetables, asparagus, sea vegetables, artichokes, and spices, are actually rather low in carbs and may be consumed on both high- and low-carb days.

Eating these meals also provides the benefit of high dietary fiber and antioxidant content. In addition to making you feel full and satiated, fiber also contains antioxidants that help slow down the aging process and battle free radical damage. In addition to increasing protein consumption and varying carbohydrates, a good carb cycle diet plan teaches you how to include necessary items in meals in ways that you really love.

5. Supports Long-Term Adherence to a Healthful Diet

Although alternative diet regimens that limit total calories may also help you lose weight, many people find that carb cycling is more effective and causes less feelings of deprivation.

A carb cycling diet has more flexibility than other diets, which might motivate individuals to remain with it since foods like grains, fruit, and legumes are allowed at least one or three times a week (often even coupled with a "cheat meal").

6. May Assist in Reducing Blood Sugar Swings and Hormonal Fluctuations

Numerous studies have shown the effectiveness of a low-carb diet as a component of a natural diabetes treatment strategy for individuals with type 2 diabetes. In certain studies, eating low-carbohydrate food has been shown to assist improve blood glucose more than low-fat diets. It has also been proven to help control blood lipid levels, BMI, and lower insulin dosages in diabetic patients.

Lower-carb diets may help decrease the risk of diabetes complications and associated risk factors including obesity and heart disease because they can minimize overeating, particularly of junk food and empty calories.

Why does limiting carbohydrates on some days raise hormone and blood sugar levels? Diets low in carbohydrates promote improvements in blood pressure management, postprandial glycemia, insulin secretion, and dyslipidemia, diabetes, and metabolic syndrome.

Periodically increasing your diet of carbohydrates and calories in general may also help prevent the levels of other important hormones, such as testosterone, progesterone, estrogen, and thyroid hormone, from falling. These hormones are essential for many other processes, including maintaining a high metabolic rate. certain individuals have been found to produce less of these hormones while on a diet or restricting their calories, particularly when paired with strenuous exercise. This suggests that certain people are more vulnerable to the hormonal changes brought on by diets due to variables such as heredity.

The science of carb cycling.

A relatively recent diet strategy is carb cycling.

The biological processes underlying the manipulation of carbohydrates provide the foundation of science.

Diets based on carb cycling have not been extensively studied in controlled trials.

Attempting to meet your body's need for calories or glucose is known as carb cycling. For instance, it supplies carbs just before or after a strenuous exercise session.

Your body replenishes its store of muscle glycogen on the high-carb days, which might enhance performance and lessen muscle breakdown.

Appetite and weight-regulating hormones, ghrelin and leptin, may also operate better during times of strategic high carbohydrate consumption.

According to reports, the low-carb days cause your body to transition to a mostly fat-based energy system, which may enhance metabolic flexibility and your body's long-term capacity to burn fat for fuel.

The regulation of insulin is a significant additional element of carb cycling.

Insulin sensitivity, an important health indicator, may be improved by the low-carb days and carbohydrate targeting around exercises.

Theoretically, this strategy may reinforce the advantages that carbs provide.

Because there isn't much direct study on carb cycling, even if the mechanics underlying it support its usage, caution is still advised. In order to determine if carb cycling is safe and effective, many additional clinical research involving human subjects are required.

Carb Cycling Meal Tips

The following advice will help you choose the healthiest carbohydrates to consume:

1. Select produce and fruits that are rich in fiber.
2. Choose dairy items such as yogurt, cheese, milk, and other low-fat options.
3. Increase your intake of legumes, such as peas, beans, and lentils.
4. Consume a lot of whole grains.
5. Refined carbohydrates, sugar additions, and highly processed meals should be avoided.

Can It Work For Fat Loss?

You may be asking yourself, "How does carb cycling work for fat loss?" at this point. Let me tell you something, science is everything. You see, your body begins using fat for energy when you ingest less carbohydrates. We refer to this as ketosis. However, if you remain in ketosis for an extended period of time, your body adjusts and the rate at which fat is burned decreases. This is the role of carb cycling. Adding high-carb days to your diet can help you maintain your body's fat-burning phase and increase your metabolism.

However, carb cycling is more than simply science. It's about the trip as well. I gained awareness of my body's demands and learnt to listen to it when I started my carb cycling journey. I came to appreciate the benefits of whole grain bread and the delights of sweet potatoes. I even developed a fresh respect for broccoli—yes, you read it correctly.

What's the finest thing, then? It is true that carb cycling is effective. I saw the pounds melt off and my energy go through the roof. The strength of carbohydrates propelled me to feel like a superhero.

Thus, my friends, if you're searching for a fun and efficient fat-loss method, consider carb cycling. Your body and taste senses will appreciate it, I promise.

What Elements Affect the Intake of Carbs?

Changing the amount of carbohydrates you eat according to your requirements and objectives is one of the most important aspects of this diet. A number of variables, including body composition, training and recovery days, medical issues, training style, and body fat percentage, might affect how much carbohydrates one consumes.

- *Body Composition:* The amount of carbohydrates you need depends on your body composition. You should probably eat less carbohydrates if you're attempting to reduce weight than if you're trying to gain muscle.
- *Days of Training and Rest:* A further factor influencing carbohydrate consumption is exercise level. You could need more carbohydrates than someone who has a sedentary lifestyle.
- *Health concerns:* You may need to modify your carbohydrate consumption if you have certain health concerns, such as metabolic syndrome or diabetes.
- *The kind of instruction:* In addition, your body may need additional carbohydrates to aid in recovery if you engage in a lot of weight training or hard activity.
- *Amount of Body Fat:* Lastly, if your body fat percentage is high, you could need less carbohydrates to meet your objectives.

Chapter 2: Getting Started with Carb Cycling

How to Set Your Carb Cycling Goals

To make sure you're headed in the right direction and getting the results you want, setting your objectives for carb cycling entails a few crucial stages. Here's a quick approach to help you choose your objectives for carb cycling:

1. *Determine your main objective:* Do you want to be in better shape, gain muscle, or become a better athlete? How you organize your carb cycling strategy will depend on your main objective.
2. *Calculate how many calories you require:* Determine how many calories you need each day depending on your age, height, weight, and degree of exercise. For a precise estimate, you might speak with a dietitian or use an online calculator.
3. *Decide on your macro goals:* You may establish your macronutrient objectives after you are aware of your calorie requirements. For carb cycling, a common rule of thumb is to ingest 1-3 grams of protein and 0.3-0.5 grams of fat for every pound of body weight, with the remaining calories coming from carbs. Adapt these figures to your objectives and tastes.
4. *Schedule your days with high and low carbs:* Plan your meals based on the number of high- and low-carb days you intend to have each week. Typically, one or two days of moderate carbohydrate eating are spaced out between three to four days of high and low carbohydrate eating.
5. *Track your development:* Track your progress by keeping an eye on your weight, body composition, and cycling or gym performance. If necessary, modify your carb cycling strategy to keep moving in the direction of your objectives.

To determine your carb consumption, visit the following link or type in the link below:

https://www.calculator.net/carbohydrate-calculator.html

Chapter 3: Breakfast

Overnight Chia Seed Pudding with Berries

Servings: 1
Cooking Time: 5 minutes
Prep Time: 5 minutes
Total Time: 10 minutes

Ingredients:

1/4 cup chia seeds
1 cup unsweetened almond milk
1/2 cup mixed berries (fresh or frozen)
1 tablespoon honey or maple syrup
1/4 teaspoon vanilla extract
Pinch of salt

Instructions:

Combine the chia seeds, almond milk, honey, vanilla essence, and a little amount of salt in a
small dish or jar. Mix well to blend.
Refrigerate the jar or dish for a minimum of two hours or overnight, covered.
Mix in a handful of mixed berries and give the pudding a thorough stir before serving.

Nutritional Information (per serving):

Calories: 290
Fat: 15g
Protein: 7g
Carbohydrates: 30g
Fiber: 12g
Sugar: 16g
Vitamin C: 20%
Calcium: 30%
Iron: 20%

Spinach and Feta Egg Muffins

Servings: 6
Cooking Time: 20 minutes
Prep Time: 10 minutes
Total Time: 30 minutes

Ingredients:

6 large eggs
1/4 cup milk
1/4 teaspoon salt
1/8 teaspoon black pepper
1 cup fresh spinach, chopped
1/3 cup crumbled feta cheese
1/4 cup diced red bell pepper
1/4 cup diced onion

Instructions:

Turn the oven on to 375°F (190°C) and spray cooking spray inside a muffin pan.
Whisk the eggs, milk, salt, and black pepper in a medium-sized bowl.
Add sliced onion, diced red bell pepper, crumbled feta cheese, and chopped spinach.
Divide the egg mixture among the muffin cups evenly.
Bake the egg muffins for 18 to 20 minutes, or until they are set and have a hint of golden color on top.
Before taking the muffins out of the pan, let them cool for a few minutes.

Nutritional Information (per serving, 1 muffin):

Calories: 90
Fat: 5g
Protein: 7g
Carbohydrates: 3g
Fiber: 0.5g
Sugar: 1g
Vitamin A: 15%
Vitamin C: 20%
Iron: 4%

Avocado Toast with Smoked Salmon

Servings: 1
Cooking Time: 5 minutes
Prep Time: 5 minutes
Total Time: 10 minutes

Ingredients:

1 slice of whole-grain bread
1/2 ripe avocado, mashed
2 oz smoked salmon
1 tablespoon chopped fresh dill
1/4 teaspoon lemon juice
Salt and pepper to taste

Instructions:

Toast the whole-grain bread piece until it reaches the desired crispness.
Over the bread, equally distribute the mashed avocado.
Place the smoked salmon on top of the avocado and top with freshly chopped dill.
After adding salt and pepper to taste, drizzle the lemon juice over the bread.

Nutritional Information (per serving):

Calories: 280
Fat: 15g
Protein: 15g
Carbohydrates: 22g
Fiber: 8g
Sugar: 2g
Vitamin C: 10%
Calcium: 6%
Iron: 8%

Greek Yogurt Parfait with Nuts and Seeds

Servings: 1
Cooking Time: 5 minutes
Prep Time: 5 minutes
Total Time: 10 minutes

Ingredients:

3/4 cup Greek yogurt
1/4 cup mixed nuts and seeds (such as almonds, walnuts, sunflower seeds, and chia seeds)
1/2 cup mixed berries (fresh or frozen)
1 tablespoon honey or maple syrup

Instructions:

Arrange the Greek yogurt, mixed nuts and seeds, and mixed berries in a glass or container.
Pour maple syrup or honey over the top.

Nutritional Information (per serving):

Calories: 350
Fat: 18g
Protein: 20g
Carbohydrates: 30g
Fiber: 5g
Sugar: 20g
Vitamin C: 20%
Calcium: 25%
Iron: 10%

Protein Pancakes with Almond Butter

Servings: 2
Cooking Time: 10 minutes
Prep Time: 5 minutes
Total Time: 15 minutes

Ingredients:

1 cup rolled oats
One scoop of protein powder, any flavor will do
1/2 teaspoon baking powder
1/4 teaspoon salt
1 large egg
1/2 cup milk
1 tablespoon almond butter
1 teaspoon coconut oil or cooking spray

Instructions:

The protein powder, baking powder, salt, and rolled oats should all be blended into a fine powder in a blender.
Blend the milk and egg in the blender until they are smooth.
Coat the pan with cooking spray or coconut oil and heat it over medium heat.
For each pancake, pour 1/4 cup of batter into the pan and cook for 2 to 3 minutes on each side, or until golden brown.
Top the pancakes with almond butter and serve.

Nutritional Information (per serving, 2 pancakes):

Calories: 330
Fat: 12g
Protein: 22g
Carbohydrates: 35g
Fiber: 5g
Sugar: 5g
Vitamin A: 6%
Calcium: 20%
Iron: 15%

Sweet Potato and Kale Hash

Servings: 2
Cooking Time: 25 minutes
Prep Time: 10 minutes
Total Time: 35 minutes

Ingredients:

1 medium sweet potato, peeled and diced
1 tablespoon olive oil
1/2 onion, diced
2 cups kale, chopped
2 large eggs
Salt and pepper to taste

Instructions:

In a large pan over medium heat, warm the olive oil. When the sweet potato is soft and starting to turn golden, add the chopped onion and simmer for another 15 to 20 minutes.
When the kale has wilted, return it to the pan with the chopped leaves and cook for a further three to four minutes.
In the hash, create two little wells and break one egg into each. When the eggs are fried to the desired doneness, cover the pan and heat for 3–4 minutes.
Serve right away after adding salt and pepper to taste.

Nutritional Information (per serving):

Calories: 260
Fat: 12g
Protein: 10g
Carbohydrates: 28g
Fiber: 4g
Sugar: 6g
Vitamin A: 250%
Vitamin C: 120%
Calcium: 10%
Iron: 10%

Low-Carb Breakfast Burritos with Egg and Cheese

Servings: 2
Cooking Time: 15 minutes
Prep Time: 10 minutes
Total Time: 25 minutes

Ingredients:

2 large eggs
2 tablespoons milk
Salt and pepper to taste
1 tablespoon olive oil
1/2 cup shredded cheese
2 low-carb tortillas
Optional toppings: salsa, avocado, or hot sauce

Instructions:

Whisk the eggs, milk, and a little amount of salt and pepper in a small bowl.
Heat the olive oil in a pan that is nonstick over medium heat. After adding the egg mixture, heat it, stirring now and then, until the eggs are cooked through and scrambled.
To let the cheese melt, scatter the shredded cheese over the eggs in the pan and cover. It should take a minute or two to complete.
For ten to fifteen seconds, reheat the low-carb tortillas in the microwave.
Spoon the egg and cheese mixture onto each of the two tortillas, then top with any additional ingredients.
Serve the tortillas right away after rolling them up.

Nutritional Information (per serving, 1 burrito):

Calories: 320
Fat: 22g
Protein: 20g
Carbohydrates: 15g
Fiber: 6g
Sugar: 2g
Vitamin A: 10%
Iron: 10%

Whole Grain Waffles with Fresh Fruit

Servings: 4
Cooking Time: 10 minutes
Prep Time: 10 minutes
Total Time: 20 minutes

Ingredients:

1 cup whole-grain flour
2 teaspoons baking powder
1/4 teaspoon salt
1 cup milk
1 large egg
2 tablespoons vegetable oil
1 cup fresh fruit (such as berries, sliced bananas, or diced peaches)
Optional toppings: maple syrup, honey, or yogurt

Instructions:

As directed by the manufacturer, preheat your waffle iron.
Mix the whole-grain flour, baking powder, and salt in a medium-sized bowl.
Beat the egg, vegetable oil, and milk together in another bowl. Mix until just blended, add the wet ingredients to the dry components.
After using cooking spray to grease the waffle iron, transfer the batter onto it. Waffles should be cooked as directed by the maker or until golden brown.
Present the waffles with your preferred extra toppings and fresh fruit on top.

Nutritional Information (per serving, 1 waffle):

Calories: 220
Fat: 9g
Protein: 7g
Carbohydrates: 29g
Fiber: 4g
Sugar: 5g
Vitamin C: 15%
Iron: 10%

Veggie-Packed Omelet

Servings: 1
Cooking Time: 10 minutes
Prep Time: 5 minutes
Total Time: 15 minutes

Ingredients:

2 large eggs
Salt and pepper to taste
1 tablespoon olive oil
1/2 cup chopped mixed vegetables (such as bell peppers, onions, mushrooms, and spinach)
1/4 cup shredded cheese

Instructions:

Whisk the eggs, salt, and pepper in a small bowl.
Heat the olive oil in a pan that is nonstick over medium heat. When the veggies are soft, add the chopped mixed vegetables and simmer for another three to four minutes.
After covering the veggies with the egg mixture, simmer for two to three minutes, or until the eggs are mostly set.
After covering one side of the omelet with shredded cheese, fold the other side over the cheese.
Simmer for one to two more minutes, or until the cheese is melted. Serve right away.

Nutritional Information (per serving):

Calories: 280
Fat: 22g
Protein: 16g
Carbohydrates: 5g
Fiber: 1g
Sugar: 2g
Vitamin A: 15%
Vitamin C: 40%
Calcium: 15%
Iron: 10%

High-Protein Oatmeal with Mixed Berries

Servings: 1
Cooking Time: 5 minutes
Prep Time: 5 minutes
Total Time: 10 minutes

Ingredients:

1/2 cup rolled oats
1 cup milk
One scoop of protein powder, any flavor will do
1/2 cup mixed berries (fresh or frozen)
1 tablespoon honey or maple syrup
Optional toppings: nuts, seeds, or nut butter

Instructions:

Mix the milk and the rolled oats in a small saucepan. Cook for 3–4 minutes, stirring periodically, over medium heat, or until the mixture has thickened and the oats are cooked.
After taking the saucepan off of the burner, thoroughly mix in the protein powder.
Spoon the oats into a bowl, then garnish with the mixed berries, honey or maple syrup, and any other toppings that you would like.

Nutritional Information (per serving):

Calories: 380
Fat: 7g
Protein: 25g
Carbohydrates: 55g
Fiber: 7g
Sugar: 20g
Vitamin C: 15%
Calcium: 30%
Iron: 15%

Turkey and Cheese Roll-Ups with Spinach

Servings: 2
Cooking Time: 5 minutes
Prep Time: 5 minutes
Total Time: 10 minutes

Ingredients:

4 slices deli turkey
2 slices cheese
1 cup fresh spinach
Optional condiments: mustard, mayo, or hummus

Instructions:

Place the turkey slices from the deli flat on a sanitized surface.
Top each piece of turkey with a slice of cheese and a generous bunch of fresh spinach.
Tightly roll the turkey and cheese, securing with a toothpick if necessary.
Serve the roll-ups with the optional condiments of your choosing.

Nutritional Information (per serving, 2 roll-ups):

Calories: 210
Fat: 12g
Protein: 21g
Carbohydrates: 3g
Fiber: 1g
Sugar: 1g
Vitamin A: 30%
Vitamin C: 10%
Calcium: 20%
Iron: 6%

Quinoa Breakfast Bowl with Nuts and Seeds

Servings: 1
Cooking Time: 15 minutes
Prep Time: 5 minutes
Total Time: 20 minutes

Ingredients:

1/2 cup cooked quinoa
1/4 cup mixed nuts and seeds (such as almonds, walnuts, sunflower seeds, and chia seeds)
1/2 cup milk
1/2 cup mixed berries (fresh or frozen)
1 tablespoon honey or maple syrup

Instructions:

Place the cooked quinoa, milk, and mixed nuts and seeds in a small saucepan. Simmer for 5 to 6 minutes, stirring often, over medium heat, or until the milk is largely absorbed.
Spoon the quinoa mixture into a bowl and drizzle with maple syrup or honey and mixed berries.

Nutritional Information (per serving):

Calories: 400
Fat: 18g
Protein: 12g
Carbohydrates: 48g
Fiber: 6g
Sugar: 18g
Vitamin C: 15%
Calcium: 15%
Iron: 15%

Cottage Cheese and Fruit Plate

Servings: 1
Cooking Time: 5 minutes
Prep Time: 5 minutes
Total Time: 10 minutes

Ingredients:

1 cup cottage cheese
1 cup mixed fruit (such as berries, sliced bananas, or diced peaches)
Optional toppings: nuts, seeds, or honey

Instructions:

Place the mixed fruit and cottage cheese onto a platter.
After adding any optional toppings of your choice, serve right away.

Nutritional Information (per serving):

Calories: 240
Fat: 2g
Protein: 24g
Carbohydrates: 32g
Fiber: 4g
Sugar: 15g
Vitamin C: 15%
Calcium: 15%
Iron: 2%

Egg and Veggie Breakfast Sandwich

Servings: 1
Cooking Time: 10 minutes
Prep Time: 5 minutes
Total Time: 15 minutes

Ingredients:

1 whole-grain English muffin
1 large egg
Salt and pepper to taste
1/2 cup chopped mixed vegetables (such as bell peppers, onions, mushrooms, and spinach)
1 slice cheese

Instructions:

Set the temperature of your toaster or oven to 375°F (190°C).
After halving the English muffin, toast it to the desired doneness.
Cook the chopped mixed veggies in a small pan over medium heat for 3 to 4 minutes, or until they are soft.
Fry the egg in a different small pan until it reaches the desired doneness. To taste, add salt and pepper for seasoning.
Place the cooked veggies, fried egg, and cheese slice on one side of the English muffin to assemble the sandwich.
Once the cheese is melted, put the prepared sandwich in the oven or toaster oven for one to two minutes.
Serve right away.

Nutritional Information (per serving):

Calories: 330
Fat: 11g
Protein: 18g
Carbohydrates: 38g
Fiber: 5g
Sugar: 2g
Vitamin A: 10%
Vitamin C: 20%

Calcium: 20%
Iron: 15%

High-Protein Smoothie Bowl

Servings: 1
Cooking Time: 5 minutes
Prep Time: 5 minutes
Total Time: 10 minutes

Ingredients:

1 cup frozen mixed berries
One scoop of your preferred flavor protein powder
1/2 cup milk
1/2 banana, sliced
Optional toppings: nuts, seeds, or shredded coconut

Instructions:

Blend together the milk, protein powder, and frozen mixed berries using a blender. Process till smooth.
Transfer the smoothie into a bowl and garnish with sliced banana and any toppings of your choice.

Nutritional Information (per serving):

Calories: 270
Fat: 4g
Protein: 24g
Carbohydrates: 35g
Fiber: 6g
Sugar: 22g
Vitamin C: 15%
Calcium: 20%
Iron: 10%

Whole Grain French Toast with Fresh Fruit

Servings: 2
Cooking Time: 10 minutes
Prep Time: 5 minutes
Total Time: 15 minutes

Ingredients:

4 slices whole-grain bread
2 large eggs
1/2 cup milk
1 teaspoon vanilla extract
1/2 teaspoon ground cinnamon
1 tablespoon butter
1 cup fresh fruit (such as berries, sliced bananas, or diced peaches)
Optional toppings: maple syrup or honey

Instructions:

Whisk the eggs, milk, ground cinnamon, and vanilla essence in a small bowl.
Make care to cover both sides of each piece of bread after dipping it into the egg mixture.
Butter should be melted in a big pan over medium heat. When the bread slices are golden brown,
add them to the pan and cook them for two to three minutes on each side.
Present the French toast garnished with optional toppings of your choice and fresh fruit.

Nutritional Information (per serving, 2 slices of French toast):

Calories: 340
Fat: 12g
Protein: 15g
Carbohydrates: 42g
Fiber: 6g
Sugar: 12g
Vitamin C: 15%
Calcium: 15%
Iron: 10%

Greek Yogurt and Granola with Mixed Berries

Servings: 1
Cooking Time: 5 minutes
Prep Time: 5 minutes
Total Time: 10 minutes

Ingredients:

1 cup Greek yogurt
1/2 cup mixed berries (fresh or frozen)
1/4 cup granola
Optional toppings: nuts, seeds, or honey

Instructions:

Arrange the Greek yogurt, granola, and mixed berries in a bowl.
After adding any optional toppings of your choice, serve right away.

Nutritional Information (per serving):

Calories: 260
Fat: 7g
Protein: 18g
Carbohydrates: 32g
Fiber: 3g
Sugar: 17g
Vitamin C: 15%
Calcium: 20%
Iron: 4%

Low-Carb Breakfast Casserole with Veggies and Cheese

Servings: 6
Cooking Time: 40 minutes
Prep Time: 10 minutes
Total Time: 50 minutes

Ingredients:

12 large eggs
1/2 cup milk
Salt and pepper to taste
2 cups chopped mixed vegetables (such as bell peppers, onions, mushrooms, and spinach)
1 cup shredded cheese
Optional toppings: fresh herbs or hot sauce

Instructions:

Heat the oven to 375°F (190°C) and coat a 9-by-13-inch baking dish with oil.
Whisk the eggs, milk, and a little amount of salt and pepper in a big bowl.
Add the shredded cheese and chopped mixed veggies and stir.
Transfer the egg mixture onto the baking dish that has been prepared, and bake for 35 to 40 minutes, or until the top of the eggs becomes golden brown.
Serve the dish hot, garnished with optional toppings if preferred.

Nutritional Information (per serving, 1/6 of the casserole):

Calories: 220
Fat: 15g
Protein: 17g
Carbohydrates: 5g
Fiber: 1g
Sugar: 2g
Vitamin A: 25%
Vitamin C: 20%
Calcium: 15%
Iron: 10%

Avocado and Egg Breakfast Salad

Servings: 1
Cooking Time: 10 minutes
Prep Time: 5 minutes
Total Time: 15 minutes

Ingredients:

1 large egg
1/2 avocado, diced
1 cup mixed greens
1/2 cup cherry tomatoes, halved
1 tablespoon olive oil
1 tablespoon balsamic vinegar
Salt and pepper to taste

Instructions:

Boil the egg for 6 to 7 minutes, or until it achieves the desired doneness, in a small pot. After letting the egg cool somewhat, peel and cut it.
Combine the chopped avocado, cherry tomatoes, and mixed greens in a bowl and toss with the balsamic vinegar and olive oil. To taste, add salt and pepper for seasoning.
Place the sliced egg on top of the salad and serve right away.

Nutritional Information (per serving):

Calories: 320
Fat: 27g
Protein: 9g
Carbohydrates: 12g
Fiber: 5g
Sugar: 4g
Vitamin A: 45%
Vitamin C: 50%
Calcium: 4%
Iron: 10%

Whole Grain Blueberry Muffins

Servings: 12
Cooking Time: 25 minutes
Prep Time: 10 minutes
Total Time: 35 minutes

Ingredients:

1 1/2 cups whole-grain flour
1/2 cup sugar
1 teaspoon baking powder
1/2 teaspoon baking soda
1/2 teaspoon salt
1 large egg
1 cup milk
1/4 cup vegetable oil
1 cup fresh blueberries

Instructions:

Adjust the oven temperature to 375°F (190°C) and place paper liners into a muffin tray.
Mix the whole-grain flour, sugar, baking soda, baking powder, and salt in a large basin.
Whisk the egg, milk, and vegetable oil in another bowl.
After adding the wet components to the dry ingredients, mix just until incorporated.
Add the fresh blueberries and fold.
Pour the batter into each muffin cup, filling it approximately 3/4 of the way.
A toothpick put into the middle of a muffin should come out clean after 20 to 25 minutes of baking.
Before serving, let the muffins cool for a few minutes.

Chapter 4: Lunch

Grilled Chicken and Veggie Bowl with Quinoa

Servings: 4
Cooking Time: 20 minutes
Prep Time: 15 minutes
Total Time: 35 minutes

Ingredients:

1 cup quinoa
2 cups water
1 lb boneless, skinless chicken breasts
1 zucchini, sliced
1 red bell pepper, sliced
1 yellow squash, sliced
1 red onion, sliced
1 tablespoon olive oil
Salt and pepper to taste
1/4 cup fresh parsley, chopped
1 lemon, juiced

Instructions:

After giving the quinoa a quick rinse in a sieve with fine mesh, move it to a medium saucepan. Add the water and bring it to a boil. Once the quinoa is cooked and the water has been absorbed, reduce the heat to low, cover, and simmer for 15 to 20 minutes.
Warm up a grill or grill pan to a temperature of medium-high.
Add salt and pepper to the chicken breasts for seasoning. The chicken should be cooked inside out by grilling it for 6 to 8 minutes on each side, or 165°F (74°C). Before slicing, take the chicken from the grill and let it rest for five minutes.
Combine the red onion, yellow squash, red bell pepper, and zucchini in a big bowl and mix with the olive oil, salt, and pepper. The veggies should be soft and faintly browned after grilling them for two to three minutes on each side.
Spoon the cooked quinoa into each of four bowls. Arrange the veggies and grilled chicken on top of each bowl.
Drizzle the bowls with the lemon juice and minced parsley. Serve right away.

Nutritional Information (per serving):

Calories: 370
Fat: 10g
Protein: 30g
Carbohydrates: 35g
Fiber: 5g
Sugar: 4g
Vitamin A: 25%
Vitamin C: 90%
Calcium: 5%
Iron: 20%

Turkey and Cheese Roll-Ups with Spinach

Servings: 4
Cooking Time: 5 minutes
Prep Time: 10 minutes
Total Time: 15 minutes

Ingredients:

8 slices of deli turkey
Four pieces of cheese, preferably cheddar or Swiss.
2 cups fresh spinach
1/2 cup thinly sliced red bell pepper
1/4 cup thinly sliced red onion
1 tablespoon Dijon mustard
Salt and pepper to taste

Instructions:

Place the turkey slices on a level, spotless surface.
Top each slice of turkey with a piece of cheese and a generous amount of red onion, bell pepper, and spinach.
Tightly roll the turkey and cheese, securing with a toothpick if necessary.
Present the roll-ups beside a dish of Dijon mustard for dunks.

Nutritional Information (per serving, 2 roll-ups):

Calories: 180
Fat: 10g
Protein: 18g
Carbohydrates: 6g
Fiber: 1g
Sugar: 2g
Vitamin A: 35%
Vitamin C: 60%
Calcium: 25%
Iron: 6%

Greek Salad with Grilled Chicken

Servings: 4
Cooking Time: 15 minutes
Prep Time: 15 minutes
Total Time: 30 minutes

Ingredients:

1 lb boneless, skinless chicken breasts
Salt and pepper to taste
1/4 cup olive oil
2 tablespoons red wine vinegar
1 tablespoon lemon juice
1 teaspoon dried oregano
4 cups romaine lettuce, chopped
1 cucumber, sliced
1 cup cherry tomatoes, halved
1/2 red onion, thinly sliced
1/2 cup Kalamata olives
1/2 cup crumbled feta cheese

Instructions:

Warm up a grill or grill pan to a temperature of medium-high.
Add salt and pepper to the chicken breasts for seasoning. The chicken should be cooked inside out by grilling it for 6 to 8 minutes on each side, or 165°F (74°C). Before slicing, take the chicken from the grill and let it rest for five minutes.
Olive oil, red wine vinegar, lemon juice, oregano, and a dash of salt and pepper should all be combined in a small basin.
Toss the romaine lettuce, cucumber, cherry tomatoes, red onion, and Kalamata olives in a big bowl.
Drizzle the salad with the dressing and toss to coat.
Arrange the salad onto four dishes. Add sliced grilled chicken and crumbled feta cheese to the top of each salad. Serve right away.

Nutritional Information (per serving):

Calories: 420
Fat: 25g

Protein: 34g
Carbohydrates: 12g
Fiber: 3g
Sugar: 5g
Vitamin A: 80%
Vitamin C: 30%
Calcium: 15%
Iron: 15%

Tuna Salad Stuffed Avocado

Servings: 4
Cooking Time: 10 minutes
Prep Time: 15 minutes
Total Time: 25 minutes

Ingredients:

2 cans (5 oz each) tuna in water, drained
1/4 cup Greek yogurt
2 tablespoons mayonnaise
1 celery stalk, finely chopped
1/4 cup red onion, finely chopped
1 tablespoon lemon juice
1 tablespoon Dijon mustard
Salt and pepper to taste
2 ripe avocados, halved and pitted

Instructions:

Tuna, Greek yogurt, mayonnaise, celery, red onion, lemon juice, Dijon mustard, and a dash of
salt and pepper should all be combined in a medium-sized dish.
Leave a 1/2-inch thick shell behind after removing part of the avocado flesh from the core of
each avocado half.
Chop the avocado flesh that was scooped and combine it carefully with the tuna mixture.
Spoon the tuna mixture into each avocado shell, and serve right away.

Nutritional Information (per serving, 1 stuffed avocado half):

Calories: 270
Fat: 18g
Protein: 16g
Carbohydrates: 12g
Fiber: 5g
Sugar: 2g
Vitamin A: 10%
Vitamin C: 20%
Calcium: 4%

Iron: 6%

Whole Grain Pasta Salad with Veggies and Feta

Servings: 6
Cooking Time: 15 minutes
Prep Time: 15 minutes
Total Time: 30 minutes

Ingredients:

8 oz whole grain pasta
1 cup cherry tomatoes, halved
1 cucumber, diced
1/2 red onion, thinly sliced
1/2 cup Kalamata olives, pitted and halved
1/2 cup crumbled feta cheese
1/4 cup chopped fresh parsley
1/4 cup olive oil
2 tablespoons red wine vinegar
1 garlic clove, minced
Salt and pepper to taste

Instructions:

Cook the whole grain pasta until al dente, following the directions on the box. After draining, rinse the pasta under cold water.
The cooked pasta, feta cheese, cherry tomatoes, cucumber, red onion, Kalamata olives, and parsley should all be combined in a big bowl.
Mix the garlic, red wine vinegar, olive oil, and a dash of salt and pepper in a small bowl.
After adding the dressing, toss to coat the spaghetti salad.
You may either serve it right away or let it rest in the fridge for a few hours before serving.

Nutritional Information (per serving):

Calories: 270
Fat: 17g

Protein: 7g
Carbohydrates: 24g
Fiber: 4g
Sugar: 3g
Vitamin A: 10%
Vitamin C: 15%
Calcium: 10%
Iron: 8%

Veggie and Hummus Sandwich on Whole Grain Bread

Servings: 2
Cooking Time: 5 minutes
Prep Time: 10 minutes
Total Time: 15 minutes

Ingredients:

4 slices whole grain bread
1/2 cup hummus
1/2 cup shredded carrots
1/2 cup sliced cucumber
1/2 cup baby spinach
1/4 cup sliced red bell pepper
Salt and pepper to taste

Instructions:

Slather each piece of bread with two tablespoons of hummus.
Arrange the shredded carrots, cucumber, red bell pepper, and baby spinach on two of the slices.
Add a dash of pepper and salt for seasoning.
Place the remaining pieces of bread, hummus side down, on top of the sandwiches.
Serve right now or store the sandwiches in plastic wrap or parchment paper for later.

Nutritional Information (per serving):

Calories: 340
Fat: 12g
Protein: 13g
Carbohydrates: 47g
Fiber: 11g
Sugar: 6g
Vitamin A: 130%
Vitamin C: 50%
Calcium: 8%
Iron: 20%

Chicken and Veggie Stir-Fry with Brown Rice

Servings: 4
Cooking Time: 20 minutes
Prep Time: 15 minutes
Total Time: 35 minutes

Ingredients:

1 cup brown rice
2 cups water
One pound of skinless, boneless chicken breasts, divided into one-inch pieces
2 tablespoons vegetable oil
2 cups broccoli florets
1 red bell pepper, sliced
1 yellow squash, sliced
1/2 cup sliced green onion
2 garlic cloves, minced
1/4 cup soy sauce
2 tablespoons honey
1 tablespoon cornstarch
Salt and pepper to taste

Instructions:

Heat the water and brown rice in a medium-sized pot until it boils. Once the rice is cooked and the water has been absorbed, reduce the heat to low, cover, and simmer for 20 to 25 minutes.
In a large pan or wok, heat the vegetable oil over medium-high heat while the rice cooks. After adding the chicken, simmer it for five to six minutes, or until it is cooked through and browned. After taking the chicken out of the pan, put it aside.
To the pan, add the broccoli, green onion, yellow squash, red bell pepper, and garlic. Cook the veggies for 4–5 minutes, or until they are crisp-tender.
Mix the cornstarch, honey, and soy sauce in a small bowl. Once the sauce has thickened, pour the mixture over the veggies and heat for one to two minutes.
Put the chicken back in the skillet and give it a good toss. To taste, add salt and pepper for seasoning.
Over the cooked brown rice, serve the stir-fried chicken and vegetables.

Nutritional Information (per serving):

Calories: 420
Fat: 12g
Protein: 32g
Carbohydrates: 47g
Fiber: 5g
Sugar: 12g
Vitamin A: 50%
Vitamin C: 120%
Calcium: 6%
Iron: 15%

Shrimp and Veggie Skewers with Quinoa

Servings: 4
Cooking Time: 15 minutes
Prep Time: 20 minutes
Total Time: 35 minutes

Ingredients:

1 cup quinoa
2 cups water
1 lb large shrimp, peeled and deveined
1 zucchini, sliced into 1/2-inch rounds
One red bell pepper, sliced into 1-inch segments
1 yellow squash, sliced into 1/2-inch rounds
1 red onion, cut into 1-inch pieces
1/4 cup olive oil
1 lemon, juiced
2 garlic cloves, minced
1 tablespoon chopped fresh parsley
Salt and pepper to taste

Instructions:

After giving the quinoa a quick rinse in a sieve with fine mesh, move it to a medium saucepan.
The water should be added and brought to a boil. Once the quinoa is cooked and the water has
been absorbed, reduce the heat to low, cover, and simmer for 15 to 20 minutes.
Warm up a grill or grill pan to a temperature of medium-high.
Thread the shrimp, red onion, yellow squash, red bell pepper, and zucchini onto skewers.
Mix the olive oil, lemon juice, parsley, garlic, and a dash of salt and pepper in a small bowl.
Drizzle the blend onto the skewers.
Cook the skewers for about 3–4 minutes on each side, or until the veggies are soft and the shrimp
is pink.
Over the cooked quinoa, serve the vegetable skewers and shrimp.

Nutritional Information (per serving):

Calories: 410
Fat: 16g

Protein: 25g
Carbohydrates: 42g
Fiber: 6g
Sugar: 5g
Vitamin A: 30%
Vitamin C: 100%
Calcium: 8%
Iron: 20%

Turkey and Cheese Lettuce Wraps

Servings: 4
Cooking Time: 5 minutes
Prep Time: 10 minutes
Total Time: 15 minutes

Ingredients:

Eight huge leaves of lettuce, such butter lettuce or romaine
8 slices deli turkey
4 slices cheese (such as Swiss or cheddar)
1 tomato, thinly sliced
1 avocado, sliced
1/4 cup thinly sliced red onion
Salt and pepper to taste

Instructions:

Spread out the lettuce leaves evenly on a sanitized surface.
Top each lettuce leaf with a slice of turkey, then a piece of cheese, a tomato, an avocado, and a
red onion.
Add a dash of pepper and salt for seasoning.
If necessary, firmly roll up the lettuce leaves and fasten with a toothpick.
Serve right away.

Nutritional Information (per serving, 2 lettuce wraps):

Calories: 220
Fat: 13g
Protein: 17g
Carbohydrates: 9g
Fiber: 4g
Sugar: 2g
Vitamin A: 60%
Vitamin C: 15%
Calcium: 20%
Iron: 6%

Grilled Veggie and Hummus Pita Pocket

Servings: 4
Cooking Time: 10 minutes
Prep Time: 15 minutes
Total Time: 25 minutes

Ingredients:

1 red bell pepper, sliced
1 yellow squash, sliced
1 zucchini, sliced
1 red onion, sliced
1 tablespoon olive oil
Salt and pepper to taste
1/4 cup hummus
4 whole grain pita pockets
1/2 cup baby spinach
1/4 cup crumbled feta cheese

Instructions:

Warm up a grill or grill pan to a temperature of medium-high.
Combine the red onion, yellow squash, zucchini, and red bell pepper in a big bowl along with the olive oil and a little salt and pepper.
The veggies should be grilling for 4–5 minutes on each side, or until they are soft and beginning to caramelize.
Divide one spoonful of hummus among the pita pockets.
Top the grilled veggies, baby spinach, and crumbled feta cheese into the pita pockets.
Serve right away.

Nutritional Information (per serving):

Calories: 270
Fat: 9g
Protein: 9g
Carbohydrates: 39g
Fiber: 6g
Sugar: 5g

Vitamin A: 40%
Vitamin C: 70%
Calcium: 10%
Iron: 15%

Whole Grain Veggie Pizza with Mozzarella

Servings: 4
Cooking Time: 15 minutes
Prep Time: 20 minutes
Total Time: 35 minutes

Ingredients:

1 whole grain pizza crust
1/2 cup marinara sauce
1 cup shredded mozzarella cheese
1 cup sliced mushrooms
1/2 cup sliced red bell pepper
1/2 cup sliced red onion
1/2 cup baby spinach
1/4 cup sliced black olives
1 tablespoon olive oil
Salt and pepper to taste
Fresh basil leaves, for garnish

Instructions:

Set the oven temperature to 425°F (220°C).
Evenly cover the whole grain pizza dough with marinara sauce.
Over the sauce, scatter the mozzarella cheese shreds.
Place the baby spinach, black olives, red bell pepper, red onion, and mushrooms on top of the cheese.
Sprinkle some salt and pepper on top of the pizza after drizzling it with olive oil.
Bake the pizza for 12 to 15 minutes, or until the cheese is bubbling and melted and the dough is golden.
Before slicing, take the pizza out of the oven and allow it to cool for a few minutes.
Serve the pizza right away after adding some fresh basil leaves as a garnish.

Nutritional Information (per serving):

Calories: 320
Fat: 15g
Protein: 13g
Carbohydrates: 35g
Fiber: 5g
Sugar: 4g
Vitamin A: 15%
Vitamin C: 40%
Calcium: 20%
Iron: 10%

Black Bean and Veggie Salad with Avocado

Servings: 4
Cooking Time: 15 minutes
Prep Time: 15 minutes
Total Time: 30 minutes

Ingredients:

One can (15 oz) of rinsed and drained black beans
1 cup cooked quinoa
1 cup cherry tomatoes, halved
1 cucumber, diced
1 red bell pepper, diced
1/2 red onion, diced
1 avocado, diced
1/4 cup chopped fresh cilantro
1/4 cup olive oil
2 tablespoons red wine vinegar
1 garlic clove, minced
Salt and pepper to taste

Instructions:

Black beans, cooked quinoa, cherry tomatoes, cucumber, red bell pepper, red onion, avocado, and cilantro should all be combined in a big bowl.
Mix the garlic, red wine vinegar, olive oil, and a dash of salt and pepper in a small bowl.
Toss to coat the black bean and vegetable salad after adding the dressing.
You may either serve it right away or let it rest in the fridge for a few hours before serving.

Nutritional Information (per serving):

Calories: 360
Fat: 18g
Protein: 11g
Carbohydrates: 41g
Fiber: 11g
Sugar: 4g
Vitamin A: 30%

Vitamin C: 70%
Calcium: 6%
Iron: 15%

Chicken and Veggie Soup with Whole Grain Crackers

Servings: 6
Cooking Time: 30 minutes
Prep Time: 15 minutes
Total Time: 45 minutes

Ingredients:

1 tablespoon olive oil
One pound of skinless, boneless chicken breasts, divided into one-inch pieces
1 onion, chopped
2 garlic cloves, minced
4 cups low-sodium chicken broth
1 can (14.5 oz) diced tomatoes, undrained
2 carrots, sliced
2 celery stalks, sliced
One cup of cleaned and sliced into one-inch pieces green beans
1 zucchini, sliced
1 teaspoon dried basil
1 teaspoon dried oregano
Salt and pepper to taste
6 whole grain crackers, for serving

Instructions:

In a large saucepan, warm the olive oil over medium heat. When the chicken is browned, sauté it for five to six minutes after adding it. After taking the chicken out of the saucepan, put it aside. Add the garlic and onion to the same saucepan. Simmer the onion for 3–4 minutes, or until it becomes tender.
Add the diced tomatoes and chicken broth. Heat the mixture until it boils.
To the pot, add the zucchini, carrots, celery, green beans, basil, and oregano. Also add the chicken back to the pot. Once the veggies are soft, reduce the heat to low, cover, and simmer for 15 to 20 minutes.

Add salt and pepper to taste while preparing the soup.
Present the chicken and vegetable soup with whole grain crackers.

Nutritional Information (per serving):

Calories: 220
Fat: 6g
Protein: 24g
Carbohydrates: 18g
Fiber: 4g
Sugar: 6g
Vitamin A: 80%
Vitamin C: 40%
Calcium: 6%
Iron: 10%

Spinach and Feta Stuffed Chicken Breast with Brown Rice

Servings: 4
Cooking Time: 30 minutes
Prep Time: 15 minutes
Total Time: 45 minutes

Ingredients:

1 cup brown rice
2 cups water
4 boneless, skinless chicken breasts
Salt and pepper to taste
1 cup fresh spinach
1/2 cup crumbled feta cheese
1 tablespoon olive oil
1 lemon, juiced
1 garlic clove, minced
1/4 cup chopped fresh parsley
1/4 teaspoon dried oregano

Instructions:

Heat the water and brown rice in a medium-sized pot until it boils. Once the rice is cooked and the water has been absorbed, reduce the heat to low, cover, and simmer for 20 to 25 minutes.
Set oven temperature to 400°F, or 200°C.
Cut the chicken breasts in half lengthwise, but not through. This is known as butterflying. Crack up the chicken breasts and sprinkle a little salt and pepper inside.
In the middle of each chicken breast, place 2 tablespoons of crumbled feta cheese and a handful of spinach. Refold the chicken so that the stuffing is enclosed.
Mix the olive oil, lemon juice, parsley, garlic, and oregano in a small bowl. Drizzle the blend onto the filled chicken breasts.
After the chicken is cooked through, place the packed chicken breasts in a baking sheet and bake for 25 to 30 minutes.
Serve the cooked brown rice beside the chicken breasts packed with spinach and feta.

Nutritional Information (per serving):

Calories: 370

Fat: 12g
Protein: 35g
Carbohydrates: 30g
Fiber: 3g
Sugar: 1g
Vitamin A: 20%
Vitamin C: 25%
Calcium: 15%
Iron: 10%

Grilled Shrimp and Veggie Skewers with Quinoa

Servings: 4
Cooking Time: 15 minutes
Prep Time: 20 minutes
Total Time: 35 minutes

Ingredients:

1 cup quinoa
2 cups water
1 lb large shrimp, peeled and deveined
1 zucchini, sliced into 1/2-inch rounds
Cut one red bell pepper into 1-inch slices.
1 yellow squash, sliced into 1/2-inch rounds
1 red onion, cut into 1-inch pieces
1/4 cup olive oil
1 lemon, juiced
2 garlic cloves, minced
1 tablespoon chopped fresh parsley
Salt and pepper to taste

Instructions:

After giving the quinoa a quick rinse in a sieve with fine mesh, move it to a medium saucepan.
The water should be added and brought to a boil. Once the quinoa is cooked and the water has
been absorbed, reduce the heat to low, cover, and simmer for 15 to 20 minutes.
Warm up a grill or grill pan to a temperature of medium-high.
Thread the shrimp, red onion, yellow squash, red bell pepper, and zucchini onto skewers.
Mix the olive oil, lemon juice, parsley, garlic, and a dash of salt and pepper in a small bowl.
Drizzle the blend onto the skewers.
Cook the skewers for about 3–4 minutes on each side, or until the veggies are soft and the shrimp
is pink.
Over the cooked quinoa, serve the grilled shrimp and vegetable skewers.

Nutritional Information (per serving):

Calories: 410
Fat: 16g

Protein: 25g
Carbohydrates: 42g
Fiber: 6g
Sugar: 5g
Vitamin A: 30%
Vitamin C: 100%
Calcium: 8%
Iron: 20%

Whole Grain Pasta with Turkey Bolognese

Servings: 6
Cooking Time: 30 minutes
Prep Time: 15 minutes
Total Time: 45 minutes

Ingredients:

12 oz whole grain pasta
1 tablespoon olive oil
1 lb ground turkey
1 onion, chopped
2 garlic cloves, minced
1 can (28 oz) crushed tomatoes
1 teaspoon dried basil
1 teaspoon dried oregano
Salt and pepper to taste
1/4 cup grated Parmesan cheese, for serving

Instructions:

Cook the whole grain pasta until al dente, following the directions on the box. After draining, put away.
Over medium heat, warm the olive oil in a large skillet. Cook the ground turkey for five to six minutes, or until browned, after adding it.
When the onion is tender, add the garlic and onion to the skillet and simmer for an additional three to four minutes.
Add the smashed tomatoes, basil, oregano, and a dash of salt and pepper after that. Once the mixture reaches a simmer, cook it for fifteen to twenty minutes, or until the sauce thickens.
Top the whole grain pasta with grated Parmesan cheese and serve with the turkey bolognese sauce.

Nutritional Information (per serving):

Calories: 380
Fat: 11g
Protein: 26g
Carbohydrates: 45g

Fiber: 9g
Sugar: 7g
Vitamin A: 15%
Vitamin C: 20%
Calcium: 10%
Iron: 15%

Veggie and Hummus Pita Pizza

Servings: 4
Cooking Time: 10 minutes
Prep Time: 15 minutes
Total Time: 25 minutes

Ingredients:

4 whole grain pita pockets
1/2 cup hummus
1 cup cherry tomatoes, halved
1 cucumber, sliced
1 red bell pepper, sliced
1/2 red onion, sliced
1/2 cup crumbled feta cheese
Salt and pepper to taste
Fresh basil leaves, for garnish

Instructions:

Set the oven temperature to 425°F (220°C).
Each pita pocket should have two tablespoons of hummus on it.
On top of the hummus, arrange the cherry tomatoes, cucumber, red bell pepper, and red onion.
Add more salt and pepper to taste and scatter the crumbled feta cheese on top of the veggies.
After arranging the pita pizzas on a baking sheet, bake them for 8 to 10 minutes, or until the cheese has melted and the pita is brown around the edges.
Before serving, take the pita pizzas out of the oven and allow them to cool for a few minutes.
Serve the vegetable and hummus pita pizzas right away after adding some fresh basil leaves as a garnish.

Nutritional Information (per serving):

Calories: 270
Fat: 10g
Protein: 11g
Carbohydrates: 36g
Fiber: 7g
Sugar: 5g

Vitamin A: 25%
Vitamin C: 60%
Calcium: 15%
Iron: 10%

Black Bean and Veggie Quesadillas

Servings: 4
Cooking Time: 10 minutes
Prep Time: 15 minutes
Total Time: 25 minutes

Ingredients:

One fifteen-ounce can of rinsed and drained black beans
1 cup shredded cheddar cheese
1 cup frozen corn, thawed
1 red bell pepper, diced
1/2 red onion, diced
1/4 cup chopped fresh cilantro
1/2 teaspoon ground cumin
Salt and pepper to taste
4 whole grain tortillas
Salsa and sour cream, for serving

Instructions:

Combine the black beans, cheddar cheese, corn, red onion, bell pepper, cilantro, cumin, and a dash of salt and pepper in a big bowl.
A big skillet should be heated to medium heat. Spoon a quarter of the black bean and vegetable mixture onto one side of a tortilla that has been placed in the pan. After folding the second half of the tortilla over the filling, fry it for two to three minutes on each side, or until the cheese has melted and the tortilla is golden.
Continue with the remaining tortillas and the combination of black beans and vegetables.
The black bean and vegetable quesadillas should be served with sour cream and salsa on the side.

Nutritional Information (per serving):

Calories: 360
Fat: 12g
Protein: 16g
Carbohydrates: 47g
Fiber: 10g
Sugar: 4g
Vitamin A: 20%
Vitamin C: 50%
Calcium: 25%
Iron: 15%

Grilled Chicken and Veggie Skewers with Brown Rice

Servings: 4
Cooking Time: 15 minutes
Prep Time: 20 minutes
Total Time: 35 minutes

Ingredients:

1 cup brown rice
2 cups water
One pound of skinless, boneless chicken breasts, divided into one-inch pieces
1 zucchini, sliced into 1/2-inch rounds
One red bell pepper, sliced into 1-inch segments
1 yellow squash, sliced into 1/2-inch rounds
1 red onion, cut into 1-inch pieces
1/4 cup olive oil
1 lemon, juiced
2 garlic cloves, minced
1 tablespoon chopped fresh parsley
Salt and pepper to taste

Instructions:

After giving the brown rice a quick rinse in a fine-mesh strainer, move it into a medium saucepan. The water should be added and brought to a boil. Once the rice is cooked and the water has been absorbed, reduce the heat to low, cover, and simmer for 20 to 25 minutes.
Warm up a grill or grill pan to a temperature of medium-high.
Thread the chicken, red onion, yellow squash, red bell pepper, and zucchini onto skewers.
Mix the olive oil, lemon juice, parsley, garlic, and a dash of salt and pepper in a small bowl.
Drizzle the blend onto the skewers.
Cook the skewers for 3–4 minutes on each side, or until the veggies are soft and the chicken is cooked through.
Serve the prepared brown rice with the grilled chicken and vegetable skewers.

Nutritional Information (per serving):

Calories: 410
Fat: 16g

Protein: 25g
Carbohydrates: 42g
Fiber: 6g
Sugar: 5g
Vitamin A: 30%
Vitamin C: 100%
Calcium: 8%
Iron: 20%

Whole Grain Spaghetti with Turkey Meatballs and Marinara

Servings: 6
Cooking Time: 30 minutes
Prep Time: 20 minutes
Total Time: 50 minutes

Ingredients:

12 oz whole grain spaghetti
1 lb ground turkey
1/2 cup breadcrumbs
1/4 cup grated Parmesan cheese
1 egg
1/4 cup chopped fresh parsley
1 teaspoon garlic powder
Salt and pepper to taste
2 cups marinara sauce
1/4 cup grated Parmesan cheese, for serving

Instructions:

Cook the whole grain spaghetti until al dente, following the directions on the box. After draining, put away.
Ground turkey, breadcrumbs, Parmesan cheese, egg, parsley, garlic powder, and a dash of salt and pepper should all be combined in a big dish. Shape the blend into meatballs measuring one inch.
A big skillet should be heated to medium heat. When the meatballs are browned and well cooked, add them to the skillet and simmer for 8 to 10 minutes.
After pouring the marinara sauce over the meatballs, cook them for ten to fifteen minutes, or until the sauce is well heated.
Serve the turkey meatballs and marinara sauce over whole grain spaghetti, garnished with grated Parmesan cheese.

Nutritional Information (per serving):

Calories: 420
Fat: 14g
Protein: 29g

Carbohydrates: 46g
Fiber: 8g
Sugar: 6g
Vitamin A: 15%
Vitamin C: 10%
Calcium: 15%
Iron: 15%

Please wait, Your Review is Very Important…

Dear Reader,

I hope this message finds you well. Thank you for choosing to read the Noom Cookbook For Beginners. Your feedback is incredibly valuable to me, and I would love to hear your thoughts on the book. Whether you've just started, are halfway through, or have finished reading, your perspective matters.

Your feedback is immensely appreciated and will help me enhance future works.

Thank you for taking the time to share your thoughts on the Noom Cookbook For Beginners. Your support means the world to me.

Happy reading!

Dr. Valerie Kennedy

Chapter 5: Dinner

Grilled Salmon with Roasted Veggies

Servings: 4
Cooking Time: 25 minutes
Prep Time: 10 minutes
Total Time: 35 minutes

Ingredients:

4 salmon filets (6 oz each)
2 tablespoons olive oil
1 teaspoon garlic powder
1 teaspoon paprika
1 teaspoon dried thyme
Salt and pepper, to taste
2 cups broccoli florets
1 red bell pepper, sliced
1 yellow bell pepper, sliced
1 zucchini, sliced
1 cup cherry tomatoes

Instructions:

Adjust the oven temperature to 400°F (200°C) and place parchment paper on a baking pan.
Combine the paprika, thyme, garlic powder, salt, and pepper in a small bowl.
After preparing the baking sheet, place the salmon filets on it and drizzle with 1 tablespoon of olive oil. Evenly sprinkle the fish with the spice mixture.
Combine the bell peppers, zucchini, broccoli, and cherry tomatoes with the remaining 1 tablespoon olive oil, salt, and pepper in a large bowl.
On the baking sheet, arrange the veggies around the salmon.
Roast the salmon for 20 to 25 minutes in a preheated oven, or until it is cooked through and flake readily with a fork.
Serve right away with a crisp salad or your preferred side dish.

Nutritional Information (per serving):

Calories: 385
Fat: 21.4g
Protein: 34.6g
Carbohydrates: 11.2g
Vitamin A: 135% DV
Vitamin C: 187% DV
Iron: 12% DV
Calcium: 6% DV

Chicken and Veggie Stir-Fry with Brown Rice

Servings: 4
Cooking Time: 25 minutes
Prep Time: 10 minutes
Total Time: 35 minutes

Ingredients:

1 cup brown rice
1 lb boneless, skinless chicken breast, cubed
1 tablespoon cornstarch
3 tablespoons low-sodium soy sauce
2 tablespoons honey
1 tablespoon rice vinegar
1 teaspoon sesame oil
1 tablespoon vegetable oil
2 cloves garlic, minced
1 tablespoon fresh ginger, grated
1 red bell pepper, sliced
1 yellow bell pepper, sliced
1 cup broccoli florets
1 cup sugar snap peas
1 cup sliced carrots
1/2 cup sliced green onions
1/4 cup chopped fresh cilantro
Salt and pepper, to taste

Instructions:

Follow the directions on the box to cook the brown rice.
Mix the cornstarch, rice vinegar, honey, soy sauce, and sesame oil in a medium-sized bowl. Toss to coat after adding the cubed chicken.
The vegetable oil should be heated over medium-high heat in a large pan or wok. Cook the ginger and garlic for one minute, stirring all the while.
When the chicken is cooked through, add it and simmer it for five to seven minutes, stirring now and again.
To the pan, add the carrots, sugar snap peas, broccoli, and bell peppers. Cook the veggies for a further five to seven minutes, or until they are crisp-tender.
Add the cilantro and green onions, then taste and adjust the seasoning with salt and pepper.

Over the cooked brown rice, serve the stir-fried chicken and vegetables.

Nutritional Information (per serving):

Calories: 421
Fat: 9.5g
Protein: 30.7g
Carbohydrates: 51.8g
Vitamin A: 121% DV
Vitamin C: 151% DV
Iron: 11% DV
Calcium: 6% DV

Turkey and Veggie Stuffed Peppers

Servings: 4
Cooking Time: 30 minutes
Prep Time: 15 minutes
Total Time: 45 minutes

Ingredients:

4 bell peppers (any color), tops removed and seeded
1 lb lean ground turkey
1 cup cooked brown rice
1 cup diced zucchini
1 cup diced mushrooms
1/2 cup diced onion
2 cloves garlic, minced
1 teaspoon dried oregano
1/2 teaspoon dried basil
Salt and pepper, to taste
1 cup shredded mozzarella cheese
1/4 cup chopped fresh parsley

Instructions:

Turn the oven on to 375°F (190°C) and brush a 9 x 13-inch baking dish with a little oil.
Cook the ground turkey in a big pan over medium heat for 5 to 7 minutes, or until browned.
Remove any extra fat.
To the skillet, add the mushrooms, zucchini, onion, garlic, basil, oregano, and salt & pepper.
Cook the veggies for a further five to seven minutes, or until they are soft.
After adding the cooked brown rice, stir it in and heat it for one to two minutes.
Fill each bell pepper with the turkey and vegetable mixture after placing them in the baking dish that has been prepared.
Preheat the oven and bake for 20 minutes.
After taking the peppers out of the oven, cover each one with shredded mozzarella cheese.
Put the peppers back in the oven and continue to bake for a further five to ten minutes, or until the cheese is bubbling and melted.
Serve the filled peppers right away after adding some chopped parsley as a garnish

Nutritional Information (per serving):

Calories: 373
Fat: 12.6g
Protein: 34.3g
Carbohydrates: 31.5g
Vitamin A: 52% DV
Vitamin C: 203% DV
Iron: 15% DV
Calcium: 19% DV

Shrimp and Veggie Skewers with Quinoa

Servings: 4
Cooking Time: 25 minutes
Prep Time: 15 minutes
Total Time: 40 minutes

Ingredients:

1 lb large shrimp, peeled and deveined
1 cup cherry tomatoes
1 red onion, cut into 1-inch pieces
1 yellow squash, cut into 1-inch pieces
1 zucchini, cut into 1-inch pieces
1/4 cup olive oil
2 cloves garlic, minced
1 tablespoon chopped fresh parsley
1 tablespoon chopped fresh basil
Salt and pepper, to taste
1 cup uncooked quinoa
2 cups water
1 lemon, cut into wedges

Instructions:

Eight wooden skewers should be soaked in water for at least ten minutes before you preheat your grill to medium-high heat.
Olive oil, garlic, parsley, basil, salt, and pepper should all be combined in a big bowl. Toss to coat. Add the shrimp, cherry tomatoes, red onion, yellow squash, and zucchini.
In alternate rows, thread the veggies and shrimp onto the skewers.
The shrimp should be pink and the veggies should be soft and slightly browned after grilling the skewers for five to seven minutes, flipping them over now and again.
Cook the quinoa per the directions on the box while the skewers are cooking.
With lemon wedges as a garnish, serve the cooked quinoa with the shrimp and vegetable skewers.

Nutritional Information (per serving):

Calories: 412

Fat: 16.1g
Protein: 27.5g
Carbohydrates: 38.3g
Vitamin A: 13% DV
Vitamin C: 52% DV
Iron: 21% DV
Calcium: 7% DV

Grilled Chicken and Veggie Bowl with Quinoa

Servings: 4
Cooking Time: 30 minutes
Prep Time: 15 minutes
Total Time: 45 minutes

Ingredients:

One pound of skinless, boneless chicken breasts, diced into 1-inch pieces
1 tablespoon olive oil
1 teaspoon garlic powder
1 teaspoon paprika
Salt and pepper, to taste
1 cup cherry tomatoes
1 red onion, cut into wedges
1 yellow squash, cut into 1-inch pieces
1 zucchini, cut into 1-inch pieces
1 cup uncooked quinoa
2 cups water
1/4 cup chopped fresh parsley
1 lemon, cut into wedges

Instructions:

Set your grill's temperature to medium-high.
Mix the olive oil, paprika, garlic powder, salt, and pepper in a big basin. Toss to coat and add the chicken, cherry tomatoes, red onion, yellow squash, and zucchini.
Swapping out components on skewers, thread chicken and veggies together.
Cook the skewers for ten to fifteen minutes, rotating them halfway through, or until the veggies are soft and have a hint of sea and the chicken is cooked through.
Cook the quinoa per the directions on the box while the skewers are cooking.
With lemon wedges and chopped parsley on top, serve the cooked quinoa with the grilled chicken and vegetable skewers.

Nutritional Information (per serving):

Calories: 391
Fat: 9.1g

Protein: 35.1g
Carbohydrates: 41.5g
Vitamin A: 15% DV
Vitamin C: 53% DV
Iron: 19% DV
Calcium: 5% DV

Whole Grain Pasta with Chicken and Veggies

Servings: 4
Cooking Time: 25 minutes
Prep Time: 10 minutes
Total Time: 35 minutes

Ingredients:

8 oz whole grain pasta
One pound of skinless, boneless chicken breast, divided into 1-inch chunks
2 tablespoons olive oil
1 teaspoon garlic powder
Salt and pepper, to taste
1 cup cherry tomatoes, halved
1 red bell pepper, sliced
1 yellow bell pepper, sliced
1 cup broccoli florets
1/4 cup grated Parmesan cheese
1/4 cup chopped fresh parsley

Instructions:

Follow the directions on the box to cook the whole grain pasta.
Heat the olive oil in a big pan over medium-high heat. When the chicken is cooked through, add it and simmer it for five to seven minutes, stirring now and again.
To coat the chicken, add the garlic powder, salt, and pepper to the pan and toss.
To the skillet, add the broccoli, bell peppers, and cherry tomatoes. Cook the veggies for a further five to seven minutes, or until they are crisp-tender.
After draining, add the cooked pasta, chicken, and vegetables to the skillet. To mix, toss.
Garnish the pasta and chicken with chopped parsley and grated Parmesan cheese and serve with vegetables.

Nutritional Information (per serving):

Calories: 493
Fat: 13.1g
Protein: 39.4g
Carbohydrates: 51.1g

Vitamin A: 68% DV
Vitamin C: 212% DV
Iron: 14% DV
Calcium: 11% DV

Turkey and Veggie Chili with Whole Grain Bread

Servings: 4
Cooking Time: 30 minutes
Prep Time: 15 minutes
Total Time: 45 minutes

Ingredients:

1 tablespoon olive oil
1 lb lean ground turkey
1 cup diced onion
2 cloves garlic, minced
1 red bell pepper, diced
1 green bell pepper, diced
One fifteen-ounce can of washed and drained kidney beans
1 (15 oz) can diced tomatoes, undrained
1 cup water
1 tablespoon chili powder
1 teaspoon ground cumin
Salt and pepper, to taste
1/4 cup chopped fresh cilantro
4 slices whole grain bread, toasted

Instructions:

In a large saucepan over medium heat, warm the olive oil. When the ground turkey is browned, add it and simmer, stirring often, for five to seven minutes.
To the saucepan, add the onion, garlic, kidney beans, chopped tomatoes, bell peppers, water, chili powder, cumin, salt, and pepper. Mix everything together.
After bringing the chili to a simmer, cook it for 20 to 25 minutes, stirring now and again, until the flavors have combined and the veggies are soft.
Accompany the turkey and vegetarian chili with a piece of toasted whole grain bread and chopped cilantro on top.

Nutritional Information (per serving):

Calories: 473
Fat: 11.9g

Protein: 35.2g
Carbohydrates: 58.2g
Vitamin A: 41% DV
Vitamin C: 122% DV
Iron: 23% DV
Calcium: 9% DV

Grilled Chicken and Veggie Skewers with Brown Rice

Servings: 4
Cooking Time: 25 minutes
Prep Time: 15 minutes
Total Time: 40 minutes

Ingredients:

One-pound chicken breasts, deboned and skinless, sliced into 1-inch cubes
1 cup cherry tomatoes
1 red onion, cut into 1-inch pieces
1 yellow squash, cut into 1-inch pieces
1 zucchini, cut into 1-inch pieces
1/4 cup olive oil
2 cloves garlic, minced
1 tablespoon chopped fresh parsley
1 tablespoon chopped fresh basil
Salt and pepper, to taste
1 cup uncooked brown rice
2 cups water
1 lemon, cut into wedges

Instructions:

Eight wooden skewers should be soaked in water for at least ten minutes before you preheat your grill to medium-high heat.
Olive oil, garlic, parsley, basil, salt, and pepper should all be combined in a big bowl. Toss to coat and add the chicken, cherry tomatoes, red onion, yellow squash, and zucchini.
Swapping out components on skewers, thread chicken and veggies together.
Cook the skewers for ten to fifteen minutes, rotating them halfway through, or until the veggies are soft and have a hint of sea and the chicken is cooked through.
Cook the brown rice as directed on the box while the skewers are cooking.
With lemon wedges on top, serve the cooked brown rice with the grilled chicken and vegetable skewers.

Nutritional Information (per serving):

Calories: 461

Fat: 18.2g
Protein: 32.1g
Carbohydrates: 42.6g
Vitamin A: 13% DV
Vitamin C: 52% DV
Iron: 15% DV
Calcium: 5% DV

Shrimp and Veggie Fried Rice

Servings: 4
Cooking Time: 25 minutes
Prep Time: 15 minutes
Total Time: 40 minutes

Ingredients:

1 cup uncooked brown rice
2 cups water
1 tablespoon olive oil
1 lb large shrimp, peeled and deveined
One cup of frozen mixed veggies (corn, carrots, and peas)
2 cloves garlic, minced
1 tablespoon grated fresh ginger
3 tablespoons low-sodium soy sauce
2 tablespoons rice vinegar
Salt and pepper, to taste
2 green onions, sliced
1/4 cup chopped fresh cilantro

Instructions:

Follow the directions on the box to cook the brown rice.
Heat the olive oil in a big pan or wok over medium-high heat. Cook the shrimp for two to three minutes, or until they are fully cooked and pink. After taking the shrimp out of the pan, put it aside.
Ginger, garlic, and frozen mixed veggies should all be added to the skillet. Simmer the veggies for three to four minutes, or until they are soft.
To the skillet, add the cooked brown rice, soy sauce, rice vinegar, salt, and pepper. Cook, stirring, for two to three minutes, or until well heated.
Add the cooked shrimp back to the skillet and mix everything together.
Garnish the shrimp and vegetable fried rice with chopped cilantro and sliced green onions.

Nutritional Information (per serving):

Calories: 391
Fat: 6.4g

Protein: 26.7g
Carbohydrates: 54.3g
Vitamin A: 35% DV
Vitamin C: 13% DV
Iron: 12% DV
Calcium: 6% DV

Turkey and Veggie Meatloaf with Roasted Sweet Potatoes

Servings: 4
Cooking Time: 50 minutes
Prep Time: 15 minutes
Total Time: 1 hour 5 minutes

Ingredients:

1 lb lean ground turkey
1 cup grated zucchini
1/2 cup grated carrot
1/2 cup grated onion
1/2 cup whole wheat breadcrumbs
1 egg
1 tablespoon Worcestershire sauce
1 teaspoon dried thyme
Salt and pepper, to taste
Peel and chop two sweet potatoes into 1-inch chunks.
1 tablespoon olive oil
1/4 cup chopped fresh parsley

Instructions:

Adjust the oven temperature to 375°F (190°C) and place parchment paper on a baking pan.
Ground turkey, zucchini, carrot, onion, breadcrumbs, egg, Worcestershire sauce, thyme, salt, and
pepper should all be combined in a big bowl. Toss to blend thoroughly.
Spoon the turkey mixture onto the baking sheet that has been preheated, then form it into a loaf.
Toss the sweet potato cubes with the olive oil, salt, and pepper in another bowl. Encircle the
meatloaf on the baking sheet with the sweet potatoes.
Place the sweet potatoes and meatloaf in the preheated oven and bake for 45 to 50 minutes, or
until the meatloaf reaches an internal temperature of 165°F (74°C).
Garnish the roasted sweet potatoes with minced parsley and serve with the turkey and vegetable
meatloaf.

Nutritional Information (per serving):

Calories: 401
Fat: 13.2g

Protein: 32.2g
Carbohydrates: 37.1g
Vitamin A: 114% DV
Vitamin C: 23% DV
Iron: 18% DV
Calcium: 7% DV

Whole Grain Veggie Pizza with Mozzarella

Servings: 4
Cooking Time: 25 minutes
Prep Time: 15 minutes
Total Time: 40 minutes

Ingredients:

1 whole grain pizza crust (12-14 inches)
1 cup pizza sauce
1 cup shredded mozzarella cheese
1 cup sliced bell peppers (assorted colors)
1 cup sliced mushrooms
1/2 cup sliced red onion
1/4 cup sliced black olives
1/4 cup chopped fresh basil
1/4 cup grated Parmesan cheese

Instructions:

Turn the oven on to 425°F (220°C) and line a baking sheet or pizza pan with parchment paper.
Leaving a 1/2-inch border all the way around the edge, spread the pizza sauce evenly over the whole grain pizza dough.
Over the sauce, scatter the mozzarella cheese shreds.
On top of the cheese, arrange the bell peppers, mushrooms, red onion, and black olives.
For 15 to 20 minutes, or until the cheese is melted and bubbling and the dough is golden brown, bake the pizza in a preheated oven.
After taking the pizza out of the oven, top it with grated Parmesan cheese and chopped basil.
Give the pizza a few minutes to cool down before slicing and serving.

Nutritional Information (per serving):

Calories: 482
Fat: 18.1g
Protein: 24.1g
Carbohydrates: 58.4g
Vitamin A: 32% DV
Vitamin C: 71% DV
Iron: 19% DV

Calcium: 28% DV

Chicken and Veggie Soup with Whole Grain Crackers

Servings: 4
Cooking Time: 30 minutes
Prep Time: 15 minutes
Total Time: 45 minutes

Ingredients:

1 tablespoon olive oil
One pound of skinless, boneless chicken breasts, diced into 1-inch pieces
1 cup diced onion
2 cloves garlic, minced
1 cup diced carrot
1 cup diced celery
1 cup frozen peas
4 cups low-sodium chicken broth
1 teaspoon dried thyme
Salt and pepper, to taste
1/2 cup whole grain crackers

Instructions:

Over medium heat, warm the olive oil in a large saucepan. Add the chicken and cook, stirring periodically, for 5 to 7 minutes, or until browned.
To the saucepan, add the thyme, chicken stock, onion, garlic, carrot, celery, peas, and salt and pepper. Mix everything together.
Once the chicken is cooked through and the veggies are soft, bring the soup to a boil and cook for 20 to 25 minutes.
Present the chicken and vegetable soup with whole grain crackers.

Nutritional Information (per serving):

Calories: 311
Fat: 9.1g
Protein: 32.5g

Carbohydrates: 23.5g
Vitamin A: 106% DV
Vitamin C: 12% DV
Iron: 12% DV
Calcium: 5% DV

Grilled Veggie and Hummus Pita Pocket

Servings: 4
Cooking Time: 25 minutes
Prep Time: 15 minutes
Total Time: 40 minutes

Ingredients:

1 cup hummus
4 whole grain pita pockets
1 red bell pepper, sliced
1 yellow bell pepper, sliced
1 zucchini, sliced
1 yellow squash, sliced
1/2 red onion, sliced
1 tablespoon olive oil
Salt and pepper, to taste
1/4 cup chopped fresh parsley
1 lemon, cut into wedges

Instructions:

Set your grill's temperature to medium-high.
Combine the olive oil, salt, and pepper with the bell peppers, red onion, zucchini, and yellow squash in a big bowl.
Slightly browned and soft, the veggies should be grilled for 10 to 15 minutes, flipping them over once or twice.
Grill the whole grain pita pockets for one to two minutes on each side.
Divide the 1/4 cup of hummus among the pita pockets.
Place the grilled veggies into the pita pockets and top with chopped parsley.
Pita pockets with hummus and grilled veggies should be served with lemon wedges on the side.

Nutritional Information (per serving):

Calories: 431
Fat: 15.2g
Protein: 14.2g
Carbohydrates: 62.7g

Vitamin A: 39% DV
Vitamin C: 152% DV
Iron: 18% DV
Calcium: 10% DV

Turkey and Veggie Stuffed Acorn Squash

Servings: 4
Cooking Time: 50 minutes
Prep Time: 15 minutes
Total Time: 1 hour 5 minutes

Ingredients:

2 acorn squash, halved and seeded
1 tablespoon olive oil
Salt and pepper, to taste
1 lb ground turkey
1 cup diced onion
2 cloves garlic, minced
1 cup diced carrot
1 cup diced celery
1 cup frozen peas
1/2 cup low-sodium chicken broth
1 teaspoon dried thyme
1/4 cup grated Parmesan cheese

Instructions:

Adjust the oven temperature to 400°F (200°C) and place parchment paper on a baking pan.
Add salt and pepper to the acorn squash after sprinkling it with olive oil on its sliced sides.
Squash should be placed cut-side down on the ready baking sheet.
Bake the squash for 30 to 35 minutes, or until it is soft, in a preheated oven.
The ground turkey should be cooked in a big pan over medium heat for five to seven minutes, turning often, until it is browned.
To the skillet, add the thyme, chicken stock, onion, garlic, carrot, celery, peas, and salt and pepper. Mix everything together.
Simmer the turkey and mixed vegetables for ten to twelve minutes, or until the veggies are soft.
After taking them out of the oven, gently flip the squash cut-side up. Top each half of the squash with the turkey and vegetable mixture.
Over each filled squash, sprinkle the grated Parmesan cheese.
Put the filled squash back in the oven and bake it for a further five to ten minutes, or until the cheese is bubbling and melted.
Serve the heated filled acorn squash with turkey and vegetables.

Nutritional Information (per serving):

Calories: 402
Fat: 14.5g
Protein: 29.8g
Carbohydrates: 38.2g
Vitamin A: 131% DV
Vitamin C: 51% DV
Iron: 17% DV
Calcium: 12% DV

Whole Grain Pasta with Chicken and Spinach

Servings: 4
Cooking Time: 25 minutes
Prep Time: 10 minutes
Total Time: 35 minutes

Ingredients:

8 oz whole grain pasta
Cut into 1-inch cubes, one pound of boneless, skinless chicken breasts
1 tablespoon olive oil
1 cup low-sodium chicken broth
1/2 cup heavy cream
4 cups fresh spinach
Salt and pepper, to taste
1/4 cup grated Parmesan cheese
1/4 cup chopped fresh parsley

Instructions:

Follow the directions on the box to cook the whole grain pasta.
In a large skillet, heat the olive oil over medium heat. Add the chicken and cook, stirring
periodically, for 5 to 7 minutes, or until browned.
To the skillet, add the heavy cream and chicken broth. After bringing the mixture to a simmer,
cook it for five to seven minutes, or until the sauce has somewhat thickened.
When the spinach has wilted, add it to the pan and simmer for two to three minutes.
To taste, add salt and pepper to the chicken and spinach to season them.
After draining, add the cooked pasta, chicken, and spinach to the skillet. To mix, toss.
Serve the whole grain pasta with chopped parsley and grated Parmesan cheese on top, along with
the chicken and spinach.

Nutritional Information (per serving):

Calories: 516
Fat: 16.8g
Protein: 41.1g
Carbohydrates: 48.1g
Vitamin A: 73% DV

Vitamin C: 21% DV
Iron: 18% DV
Calcium: 16% DV

Grilled Chicken and Veggie Skewers with Quinoa Salad

Servings: 4
Cooking Time: 25 minutes
Prep Time: 15 minutes
Total Time: 40 minutes

Ingredients:

One pound of skinless, boneless chicken breasts, sliced into 1-inch chunks
1 cup cherry tomatoes
1 red onion, cut into 1-inch pieces
1 yellow squash, cut into 1-inch pieces
1 zucchini, cut into 1-inch pieces
1 tablespoon olive oil
Salt and pepper, to taste
1 cup uncooked quinoa
2 cups water
1/4 cup chopped fresh parsley
1 lemon, cut into wedges

Instructions:

Eight wooden skewers should be soaked in water for at least ten minutes before you preheat your grill to medium-high heat.
Alternately thread the chicken, cherry tomatoes, red onion, yellow squash, and zucchini onto the skewers.
Season the skewers with salt and pepper after brushing them with olive oil.
Cook the skewers for ten to fifteen minutes, rotating them halfway through, or until the veggies are soft and have a hint of sea and the chicken is cooked through.
Cook the quinoa per the directions on the box while the skewers are cooking.
The cooked quinoa, parsley, and one lemon wedge's juice should all be combined in a big dish.
To taste, add salt and pepper for seasoning.
With lemon wedges on top, serve the quinoa salad with the grilled chicken and vegetable skewers.

Nutritional Information (per serving):

Calories: 441

Fat: 11.9g
Protein: 35.2g
Carbohydrates: 49.6g
Vitamin A: 13% DV
Vitamin C: 52% DV
Iron: 17% DV
Calcium: 6% DV

Whole Grain Veggie Pizza with Feta and Arugula

Servings: 4
Cooking Time: 25 minutes
Prep Time: 15 minutes
Total Time: 40 minutes

Ingredients:

1 whole grain pizza crust (12-14 inches)
1 cup pizza sauce
1 cup shredded mozzarella cheese
1 cup sliced bell peppers (assorted colors)
1 cup sliced mushrooms
1/2 cup sliced red onion
1/4 cup sliced black olives
1/4 cup crumbled feta cheese
2 cups fresh arugula
1 lemon, cut into wedges

Instructions:

Turn the oven on to 425°F (220°C) and line a baking sheet or pizza pan with parchment paper.
Leaving a 1/2-inch border all the way around the edge, spread the pizza sauce evenly over the whole grain pizza dough.
Over the sauce, scatter the mozzarella cheese shreds.
On top of the cheese, arrange the bell peppers, mushrooms, red onion, and black olives.
For 15 to 20 minutes, or until the cheese is melted and bubbling and the dough is golden brown, bake the pizza in a preheated oven.
Take the pizza out of the oven and top it with some freshly chopped arugula and crumbled feta cheese.
Present the whole grain vegetable pizza topped with lemon wedges, feta, and arugula.

Nutritional Information (per serving):

Calories: 411
Fat: 15.1g
Protein: 18.1g
Carbohydrates: 52.4g

Vitamin A: 27% DV
Vitamin C: 66% DV
Iron: 16% DV
Calcium: 21% DV

Turkey and Veggie Stuffed Peppers

Servings: 4
Cooking Time: 40 minutes
Prep Time: 15 minutes
Total Time: 55 minutes

Ingredients:

4 large bell peppers, halved and seeded
1 lb lean ground turkey
1 cup diced onion
2 cloves garlic, minced
1 cup diced carrot
1 cup diced celery
1 cup frozen peas
1 cup cooked brown rice
1 tablespoon Worcestershire sauce
Salt and pepper, to taste
1/4 cup grated Parmesan cheese

Instructions:

Adjust the oven temperature to 375°F (190°C) and place parchment paper on a baking pan.
Place the bell pepper halves cut-side up onto the baking sheet that has been preheated.
The ground turkey should be cooked in a big pan over medium heat for five to seven minutes, turning often, until it is browned.
To the pan, add the brown rice, Worcestershire sauce, onion, garlic, carrot, celery, peas, and salt and pepper. Mix everything together.
Simmer the turkey and mixed vegetables for ten to twelve minutes, or until the veggies are soft.
Place a filling of turkey and vegetable mixture on each side of a bell pepper.
Over each filled pepper, sprinkle the grated Parmesan cheese.
For 20 to 25 minutes, or until the peppers are soft and the cheese is melted and bubbling, bake the filled peppers in a preheated oven.
Warm up the stuffed peppers with turkey and vegetables.

Nutritional Information (per serving):

Calories: 324

Fat: 9.1g
Protein: 27.5g
Carbohydrates: 34.3g
Vitamin A: 132% DV
Vitamin C: 223% DV
Iron: 14% DV
Calcium: 11% DV

Whole Grain Veggie Lasagna

Servings: 4
Cooking Time: 50 minutes
Prep Time: 15 minutes
Total Time: 1 hour 5 minutes

Ingredients:

8 whole grain lasagna noodles
1 tablespoon olive oil
1 cup diced onion
2 cloves garlic, minced
1 cup diced carrot
1 cup diced celery
1 cup frozen peas
1 (15 oz) container part-skim ricotta cheese
2 cups shredded mozzarella cheese
1 egg
1/4 cup chopped fresh parsley
Salt and pepper, to taste
2 cups low-sodium tomato sauce
1/4 cup grated Parmesan cheese

Instructions:

Turn the oven on to 375°F (190°C) and brush a 9 x 13-inch baking dish with a little oil.
As directed on the box, cook the whole grain lasagna noodles; drain and leave aside.
In a large pan over medium heat, warm the olive oil. Add the peas, carrot, celery, onion, and garlic. Simmer the veggies for ten to twelve minutes, or until they are soft.
Ricotta cheese, egg, parsley, salt, and pepper, along with one cup of shredded mozzarella cheese, should all be combined in a medium-sized bowl. Blend well.
Line the bottom of the baking dish with half of the tomato sauce.
If necessary, gently overlap 4 lasagna noodles while placing them over the sauce.
Place half of the vegetable mixture on top of the noodles after spreading half of the ricotta mixture over them.
With the remaining noodles, ricotta mixture, and veggie combination, repeat the layering process.
Cover the lasagna with the remaining tomato sauce and top with the remaining 1 cup of shredded mozzarella and grated Parmesan cheese.

Bake the dish for thirty minutes with the foil covering it. After removing the foil, bake for a further ten to fifteen minutes, or until the cheese is bubbling and melted.

Before slicing and serving, let the whole grain vegetable lasagna cool for ten minutes.

Grilled Veggie and Hummus Wrap

Servings: 4
Cooking Time: 15 minutes
Prep Time: 15 minutes
Total Time: 30 minutes

Ingredients:

1 tablespoon olive oil
1 zucchini, sliced
1 yellow squash, sliced
1 red bell pepper, sliced
1 yellow bell pepper, sliced
Salt and pepper, to taste
4 whole grain wraps
1 cup hummus
1 cup shredded lettuce
1/2 cup crumbled feta cheese
1 lemon, cut into wedges

Instructions:

Set your grill's temperature to medium-high.
Combine the olive oil, salt, and pepper with the zucchini, yellow squash, red bell pepper, and yellow bell pepper in a big bowl.
Grill the veggies until they are soft and gently browned, about 5 to 7 minutes, turning them over once.
Grill the whole grain wrappers for one to two minutes on each side to reheat them.
On each wrapper, spread 1/4 cup of hummus.
Top the grilled veggies with crumbled feta cheese, shredded lettuce, and wraps.
Present the hummus and grilled vegetable wraps beside lemon wedges.

Nutritional Information (per serving):

Calories: 451
Fat: 19.3g
Protein: 14.2g
Carbohydrates: 58.2g

Vitamin A: 45% DV
Vitamin C: 131% DV
Iron: 17% DV
Calcium: 13% DV

Chapter 6: Snacks and Smoothies

Greek Yogurt with Mixed Berries and Nuts

Servings: 1
Cooking Time: N/A
Prep Time: 5 minutes
Total Time: 5 minutes

Ingredients:

3/4 cup Greek yogurt
Half a cup of mixed berries, including blueberries, blackberries, and raspberries
2 tablespoons chopped mixed nuts (such as almonds, walnuts, and pecans)
1 teaspoon honey (optional)

Instructions:

Place the Greek yogurt in a dish as the foundation.
Evenly distribute the mixed berries over the yogurt.
Over the berries, scatter the chopped mixed nuts.
If desired, drizzle with honey to provide even more sweetness.
Savor your mixed berries and nuts with Greek yogurt!

Nutritional Information (per serving):

Calories: 240
Fat: 9.3g
Protein: 16.3g
Carbohydrates: 22.7g
Vitamin A: 1% DV
Vitamin C: 4% DV
Calcium: 24% DV
Iron: 5% DV

Apple Slices with Almond Butter

Servings: 1
Cooking Time: N/A
Prep Time: 5 minutes
Total Time: 5 minutes

Ingredients:

1 medium apple, cored and sliced
2 tablespoons almond butter

Instructions:

After cleaning and core the apple, cut it into wedges.
On a platter, arrange the apple slices.
Almond butter should be spooned into a little dish or other container.
Present the apple slices with almond butter so that they may be dipped. Savor your almond
butter-topped apple slices!

Nutritional Information (per serving):

Calories: 225
Fat: 12.9g
Protein: 6.2g
Carbohydrates: 27.8g
Vitamin A: 1% DV
Vitamin C: 11% DV
Calcium: 6% DV
Iron: 4% DV

Whole Grain Crackers with Hummus and Veggies

Servings: 1
Cooking Time: N/A
Prep Time: 5 minutes
Total Time: 5 minutes

Ingredients:

10 whole grain crackers
1/4 cup hummus
1/2 cup sliced mixed vegetables (such as cucumber, bell pepper, and carrot)

Instructions:

Place all of the grain crackers on a platter.
The hummus should be spooned into a little dish or container.
Cut the mixed veggies into small pieces using a sharp knife.
Present the crackers beside the veggies and hummus for drizzling. Enjoy your veggies and hummus with whole grain crackers!

Nutritional Information (per serving):

Calories: 203
Fat: 7.5g
Protein: 8.1g
Carbohydrates: 27.7g
Vitamin A: 51% DV
Vitamin C: 22% DV
Calcium: 5% DV
Iron: 11% DV

Mixed Berry and Spinach Smoothie

Servings: 1
Cooking Time: N/A
Prep Time: 5 minutes
Total Time: 5 minutes

Ingredients:

1 cup mixed berries (such as raspberries, blueberries, and blackberries)
1 cup fresh spinach
1/2 cup Greek yogurt
1/2 cup unsweetened almond milk
1 teaspoon honey (optional)

Instructions:

In a blender, combine the almond milk, Greek yogurt, spinach, and mixed berries.
To get the right consistency, add more almond milk if necessary and blend the ingredients until they are smooth.
After tasting the smoothie, taste it again and add more honey if you'd like.
Enjoy the Mixed Berry and Spinach Smoothie after pouring it into a glass!

Nutritional Information (per serving):

Calories: 187
Fat: 2.3g
Protein: 13.3g
Carbohydrates: 32.5g
Vitamin A: 55% DV
Vitamin C: 38% DV
Calcium: 27% DV
Iron: 8% DV

Turkey and Cheese Roll-Ups with Spinach

Servings: 1
Cooking Time: N/A
Prep Time: 5 minutes
Total Time: 5 minutes

Ingredients:

1 whole wheat tortilla (8-inch)
2 tablespoons cream cheese, softened
1/4 cup fresh spinach leaves
2 oz deli turkey breast, sliced
1 oz Swiss cheese, sliced

Instructions:

Place the whole wheat tortilla in a flat, tidy heap.
Over the tortilla, equally distribute the cream cheese.
Leaving approximately an inch of space around the borders, arrange the fresh spinach leaves on top of the cream cheese.
Place the pieces of Swiss cheese and deli turkey on top of the spinach.
Tuck the items into the tortilla as you carefully wrap it.
Enjoy the Turkey and Cheese Roll-Ups with Spinach after slicing them into 1-inch pieces!

Nutritional Information (per serving):

Calories: 340
Fat: 17.6g
Protein: 21.4g
Carbohydrates: 25.7g
Vitamin A: 13% DV
Vitamin C: 6% DV
Calcium: 27% DV
Iron: 11% DV

High-Protein Oatmeal with Mixed Berries

Servings: 1
Cooking Time: 5 minutes
Prep Time: 2 minutes
Total Time: 7 minutes

Ingredients:

1/2 cup rolled oats
1 cup water
Mixture of 1/2 cup berries, including blackberries, blueberries, and raspberries
1/4 cup Greek yogurt
1 tablespoon chopped mixed nuts (such as almonds, walnuts, and pecans)

Instructions:

The rolled oats and water should be combined in a small pot. After bringing to a boil, lower the heat, cover, and simmer, stirring periodically, for three to five minutes, or until the oats are soft and the mixture has thickened.
After cooking, transfer the oatmeal to a bowl.
Add the chopped mixed nuts, Greek yogurt, and mixed berries on top of the oats.
Savor your Mixed Berries and High-Protein Oatmeal!

Nutritional Information (per serving):

Calories: 288
Fat: 8.5g
Protein: 13.5g
Carbohydrates: 41.7g
Vitamin A: 1% DV
Vitamin C: 10% DV
Calcium: 12% DV
Iron: 14% DV

Banana and Peanut Butter Roll-Ups

Servings: 1
Cooking Time: N/A
Prep Time: 5 minutes
Total Time: 5 minutes

Ingredients:

1 whole wheat tortilla (8-inch)
1 tablespoon peanut butter
1 medium banana, peeled

Instructions:

Place the whole wheat tortilla in a flat, tidy heap.
Over the tortilla, evenly distribute the peanut butter.
Lay the banana peel sideways on one tortilla edge.
Tuck the banana inside the tortilla as you firmly roll it.
Enjoy the Banana and Peanut Butter Roll-Ups after slicing them into 1-inch pieces!

Nutritional Information (per serving):

Calories: 278
Fat: 10.3g
Protein: 7.9g
Carbohydrates: 42.3g
Vitamin A: 1% DV
Vitamin C: 11% DV
Calcium: 5% DV
Iron: 9% DV

Mixed Berry and Greek Yogurt Parfait

Servings: 1
Cooking Time: N/A
Prep Time: 5 minutes
Total Time: 5 minutes

Ingredients:

3/4 cup Greek yogurt
Half a cup of mixed berries, including blackberries, blueberries, and raspberries
2 tablespoons granola
1 teaspoon honey (optional)

Instructions:

In a glass or jar, add a layer of Greek yogurt to the bottom.
Spread some mixed berries over the yogurt.
Sprinkle granola over the berries.
Repeat the layers until you reach the top of the glass or jar.
Drizzle with honey if desired for added sweetness.
Enjoy your Mixed Berry and Greek Yogurt Parfait!

Nutritional Information (per serving):

Calories: 225
Fat: 5.3g
Protein: 16.8g
Carbohydrates: 30.3g
Vitamin A: 1% DV
Vitamin C: 12% DV
Calcium: 23% DV
Iron: 3% DV

Whole Grain Toast with Avocado and Egg

Servings: 1
Cooking Time: 10 minutes
Prep Time: 5 minutes
Total Time: 15 minutes

Ingredients:

1 slice whole grain bread
1/2 avocado, pitted and peeled
1 large egg
Salt and pepper, to taste
Pinch of red pepper flakes (optional)

Instructions:

Toast the whole grain bread until it reaches the desired crispness.
Mash the avocado with a fork in a small bowl while the bread is browning.
Prepare the egg as you would want it to be cooked—fried, scrambled, or poached.
Toast the bread and then spread the mashed avocado on it.
Top the avocado with the cooked egg.
Add salt, pepper, and red pepper flakes (if using) for seasoning.
Savor your whole grain toast with egg and avocado!

Nutritional Information (per serving):

Calories: 253
Fat: 15.2g
Protein: 9.5g
Carbohydrates: 20.2g
Vitamin A: 8% DV
Vitamin C: 11% DV
Calcium: 3% DV
Iron: 10% DV

Veggie and Hummus Pita Pocket

Servings: 1
Cooking Time: N/A
Prep Time: 5 minutes
Total Time: 5 minutes

Ingredients:

1 whole wheat pita pocket
1/4 cup hummus
1/2 cup mixed vegetables (such as cucumber, bell pepper, and carrot), sliced or chopped
1 oz feta cheese, crumbled
Fresh parsley, chopped (optional)

Instructions:

If preferred, you may use the oven or microwave to reheat the whole wheat pita pocket.
Slice open the pita pocket by cutting it in half.
Inside the pockets, equally distribute the hummus.
Spoon the blended veggies and feta cheese crumbles into the pockets.
Garnish with freshly chopped parsley, if desired.
Savor your pita pocket with veggies and hummus!

Nutritional Information (per serving):

Calories: 282
Fat: 10.5g
Protein: 12.2g
Carbohydrates: 36.6g
Vitamin A: 12% DV
Vitamin C: 42% DV
Calcium: 15% DV
Iron: 15% DV

High Protein Smoothie Bowl Recipe

Ingredients:

100g frozen acai
1 cup frozen mixed berries
1 frozen banana
1 cup non-dairy Greek-style yogurt
1/2 cup soy milk
2 servings vegan protein powder
1/2 teaspoon cinnamon
1 tablespoon chia seeds
1 tablespoon flax seeds
Toppings of your choice (e.g., fresh fruit, granola, coconut flakes, etc.)

Instructions:

The frozen acai, mixed berries, banana, yogurt, soy milk, protein powder, cinnamon, chia seeds,
and flax seeds should all be combined in a high-speed blender.
To get the right consistency, add more soy milk if necessary and blend until smooth and creamy.
Transfer the smoothie into a bowl and garnish with your preferred ingredients.
Savor your Smoothie Bowl with High Protein!

Nutritional Information (per serving):

Calories: 425
Fat: 11.5g
Protein: 36g
Carbohydrates: 49.2g
Fiber: 14.2g
Calcium: 35% DV
Iron: 22% DV

Whole Grain Blueberry Muffins

Servings: 12
Cooking Time: 25 minutes
Prep Time: 15 minutes
Total Time: 40 minutes

Ingredients:

1 cup whole wheat flour
1 cup rolled oats
1/2 cup brown sugar
2 teaspoons baking powder
1/2 teaspoon baking soda
1/2 teaspoon salt
1 cup low-fat milk
1/4 cup vegetable oil
1 large egg
1 teaspoon vanilla extract
1 cup fresh blueberries

Instructions:

Set oven temperature to 400°F, or 200°C. Use cooking spray or paper liners to line a muffin tray.
Combine the rolled oats, brown sugar, baking soda, baking powder, and whole wheat flour in a large basin.
Mix the egg, vegetable oil, milk, and vanilla extract in another dish.
Mix until just mixed, pour the wet components into the dry ingredients.
Fold in the blueberries gently.
Using a spatula, evenly distribute the batter into the muffin cups.
A toothpick put into the middle of a muffin should come out clean after 20 to 25 minutes of baking.
After a few minutes, let the muffins cool in the pan before moving them to a wire rack to finish cooling.

Nutritional Information (per serving):

Calories: 156
Fat: 6.2g

Protein: 3.4g
Carbohydrates: 22.8g
Fiber: 2.2g
Sugar: 10.3g
Calcium: 6% DV
Iron: 6% DV

Cottage Cheese and Fruit Plate

Servings: 1
Cooking Time: N/A
Prep Time: 5 minutes
Total Time: 5 minutes

Ingredients:

1/2 cup cottage cheese
Half a cup of mixed berries, including blueberries, blackberries, and raspberries
1/2 banana, sliced
1 kiwi, peeled and sliced
1 tablespoon honey

Instructions:

Incorporate the cottage cheese into a small bowl.
Place the kiwi, banana, and mixed berries in a circular pattern around the cottage cheese.
Over the fruit and cottage cheese, drizzle some honey.
Savor the Fruit and Cottage Cheese Plate!

Nutritional Information (per serving):

Calories: 245
Fat: 3.4g
Protein: 14.7g
Carbohydrates: 43.6g
Fiber: 6.5g
Sugar: 30.3g
Calcium: 11% DV
Vitamin C: 91% DV
Iron: 5% DV

Peanut Butter and Banana Smoothie

Servings: 1
Cooking Time: N/A
Prep Time: 5 minutes
Total Time: 5 minutes

Ingredients:

1 banana, peeled and frozen
1/2 cup almond milk
1 tablespoon peanut butter
1/4 teaspoon ground cinnamon
1/2 teaspoon honey (optional)
1/4 cup ice

Instructions:

The frozen banana, almond milk, peanut butter, ground cinnamon, honey (if used), and ice
should all be combined in a blender.
Blend till creamy and smooth.
Enjoy the Peanut Butter and Banana Smoothie after pouring it into a glass!

Nutritional Information (per serving):

Calories: 233
Fat: 10.7g
Protein: 6.2g
Carbohydrates: 32.4g
Fiber: 4.1g
Sugar: 18.7g
Calcium: 12% DV
Iron: 7% DV

Whole Grain Energy Bites with Nuts and Seeds

Servings: 12
Cooking Time: N/A
Prep Time: 15 minutes
Total Time: 15 minutes

Ingredients:

1 cup rolled oats
1/2 cup almond butter
1/4 cup honey
1/4 cup chia seeds
Diced nuts (almonds, walnuts, or pecans) to 1/4 cup
1/4 cup mixed seeds (such as sunflower, pumpkin, or sesame)
1/4 cup dried fruit (such as cranberries, raisins, or chopped dates)
1/2 teaspoon ground cinnamon
1/4 teaspoon salt

Instructions:

The rolled oats, almond butter, honey, chia seeds, chopped almonds, mixed seeds, dried fruit, ground cinnamon, and salt should all be combined in a big dish.
Roll the mixture into 1-inch balls and transfer to a baking sheet covered with paper.
To firm up, place the Whole Grain Energy Bites in the refrigerator for at least half an hour.
For up to a week, keep the energy bites refrigerated in an airtight container.

Nutritional Information (per serving):

Calories: 174
Fat: 10.1g
Protein: 4.8g
Carbohydrates: 17.7g
Fiber: 3.1g
Sugar: 8.2g
Calcium: 8% DV
Iron: 8% DV

Turkey and Cheese Lettuce Wraps

Servings: 1
Cooking Time: N/A
Prep Time: 10 minutes
Total Time: 10 minutes

Ingredients:

3 large lettuce leaves (such as romaine or butter lettuce)
2 oz deli turkey breast, sliced
1 oz Swiss cheese, sliced
1/4 avocado, pitted and sliced
1/4 cup shredded carrot
1 tablespoon honey mustard

Instructions:

On a spotless surface, arrange the lettuce leaves flat.
Arrange the shredded carrot, avocado, Swiss cheese, and turkey slices among the lettuce leaves.
Drizzle honey mustard over each lettuce wrap.
If necessary, use toothpicks to fasten the lettuce wraps after rolling them up.
Savor your Lettuce Wraps with Turkey and Cheese!

Nutritional Information (per serving):

Calories: 216
Fat: 11.4g
Protein: 18.2g
Carbohydrates: 11.2g
Fiber: 3.2g
Sugar: 5.8g
Calcium: 16% DV
Iron: 7% DV

Mixed Berry and Spinach Smoothie

Servings: 1
Cooking Time: N/A
Prep Time: 5 minutes
Total Time: 5 minutes

Ingredients:

1 cup mixed berries (such as raspberries, blueberries, and blackberries)
1 cup fresh spinach
1/2 cup Greek yogurt
1/2 cup almond milk
1/2 teaspoon honey (optional)
1/4 cup ice

Instructions:

Blend together the spinach, Greek yogurt, almond milk, mixed berries, honey (if using), and ice
in a blender.
Blend till creamy and smooth.
Enjoy the Mixed Berry and Spinach Smoothie after pouring it into a glass!

Nutritional Information (per serving):

Calories: 157
Fat: 2.1g
Protein: 9.3g
Carbohydrates: 26.2g
Fiber: 6.2g
Sugar: 17.2g
Calcium: 19% DV
Iron: 9% DV

Whole Grain Crackers with Cheese and Turkey

Servings: 1
Cooking Time: N/A
Prep Time: 5 minutes
Total Time: 5 minutes

Ingredients:

10 whole grain crackers
2 oz deli turkey breast, sliced
1 oz cheddar cheese, sliced
1/2 cup cucumber slices
1 tablespoon Dijon mustard

Instructions:

On a spotless surface, arrange the whole grain crackers.
Place a slice of turkey, a slice of cheddar cheese, and a slice of cucumber on top of each cracker.
Over each cracker, drizzle some Dijon mustard.
Savor your Turkey and Cheese with Whole Grain Crackers!

Nutritional Information (per serving):

Calories: 267
Fat: 13.3g
Protein: 16.2g
Carbohydrates: 21.5g
Fiber: 3.1g
Sugar: 1.2g
Calcium: 19% DV
Iron: 11% DV

Greek Yogurt and Granola with Mixed Berries

Servings: 1
Cooking Time: N/A
Prep Time: 5 minutes
Total Time: 5 minutes

Ingredients:

3/4 cup Greek yogurt
Half a cup of mixed berries, including blueberries, blackberries, and raspberries
1/4 cup granola
1 teaspoon honey (optional)

Instructions:

Place the Greek yogurt in a dish as the foundation.
Sprinkle the granola and mixed berries over the yogurt.
If desired, drizzle with honey to provide even more sweetness.
Savor your Granola and Greek Yogurt with Mixed Berries!

Nutritional Information (per serving):

Calories: 232
Fat: 4.5g
Protein: 14.8g
Carbohydrates: 33.1g
Fiber: 3.8g
Sugar: 20.7g
Calcium: 19% DV
Iron: 5% DV

Veggie and Hummus Sandwich on Whole Grain Bread

Servings: 1
Cooking Time: N/A
Prep Time: 5 minutes
Total Time: 5 minutes

Ingredients:

2 slices whole grain bread
2 tablespoons hummus
1/4 cup sliced cucumber
1/4 cup sliced bell pepper
1/4 cup shredded carrot
1/4 avocado, pitted and sliced
1/4 cup spinach leaves
Salt and pepper, to taste

Instructions:

Toast the whole grain bread until it reaches the desired crispness.
Every bread piece should have an equal layer of hummus on one side.
Arrange the bell pepper, cucumber, avocado, carrot, and spinach leaves on one piece of bread.
To taste, add salt and pepper for seasoning.
Place the last piece of bread, hummus side down, on top.
Enjoy your Whole Grain Bread Veggie and Hummus Sandwich after cutting it in half!

Nutritional Information (per serving):

Calories: 376
Fat: 16.2g
Protein: 11.8g
Carbohydrates: 49.7g
Fiber: 12.1g
Sugar: 5.6g
Calcium: 11% DV
Iron: 22% DV

Chapter 7: Exercise Plan

This fitness program for carb cycling combines strength training, flexibility, and cardiovascular activities. To get the best effects, the exercises should be done on the proper carb-cycling days.

High-Carb Days (2-3 days per week):

Use the additional energy from the carbohydrates to your advantage by concentrating on high-intensity exercises on days when you're eating a lot of them.

➤ *Cardio:* Engage in high-intensity interval training (HIIT) or other high-intensity cardio workouts, such as swimming, cycling, or running, for 30 to 45 minutes.
➤ *Strengthening Exercise:* Perform a full-body strength training program that includes movements such as planks, rows, lunges, push-ups, and squats. For every exercise, aim for three sets of 10–12 repetitions, with a one-minute break in between.
➤ *Flexibility:* To increase flexibility and promote healing, spend ten to fifteen minutes stretching or doing mild yoga after your exercise.

Moderate-Carb Days (2-3 days per week):

To maintain your level of fitness and to keep burning calories, concentrate on moderate-intensity exercises on days with modest carbohydrate intake.

➤ *Cardio:* Engage in 45–60 minutes of steady-state aerobic activity, such as moderate-intensity running, cycling, or utilizing an elliptical machine.
➤ *Strength Training:* Perform a split-body strength training regimen, concentrating on exercises for the upper body one day and the lower body the next. For every exercise, aim for three sets of 10–12 repetitions, with a one-minute break in between.
➤ *Flexibility:* To increase flexibility and promote healing, spend ten to fifteen minutes stretching or doing mild yoga after your exercise.

Low-Carb Days (1-2 days per week):

Try to stick to lower-intensity exercise on low-carb days in order to maintain energy and aid in fat reduction.

➤ *Cardio:* Engage in 20–30 minutes of steady-state, low-intensity aerobic activity, such as brisk walking, easy cycling, or leisurely swimming.

➤ *Strength Training:* Work out your whole body in a circuit training program, doing each exercise with little to no break in between. For every exercise, aim for 2-3 sets of 10–12 repetitions, with a 30-second break in between.

➤ *Flexibility:* To increase flexibility and promote healing, spend ten to fifteen minutes stretching or doing mild yoga after your exercise.

Rest Days (1-2 days per week):

It is imperative that you take rest days so that your body can repair and grow new muscle. Make the most of these days by concentrating on easy exercises like mild yoga, stretching, and walking.

In order to support your workout regimen and general health, don't forget to drink lots of water, eat a balanced diet, and get plenty of sleep.

Sample Exercise Plan

Day 1:

30 minutes of vigorous riding or walking
Bodyweight squats: three sets of ten to twelve repetitions
Three sets of ten to twelve wall push-ups
3 sets of 10–12 repetitions using a resistance band for sitting rows
Stretching for ten minutes, with an emphasis on the shoulders, chest, and hamstrings

Day 2:

Swimming or water aerobics for thirty minutes
Step-ups: 3 sets of 10–12 repetitions (on a bench or step)
Three sets of dumbbell shoulder presses (10–12 repetitions)
Three sets of dumbbell bicep curls, 10–12 repetitions each
Stretching for ten minutes, with an emphasis on the quadriceps, hips, and calves

Day 3: Rest and recovery day

Day 4:

30 minutes of exercises or dance
Three sets of ten to twelve lunge repetitions, switching legs
3 sets of 10–12 repetitions of bench or chair triceps dips
Three sets of ten to twelve repetitions of dumbbell bent-over rows
Stretching for ten minutes with an emphasis on the arms, chest, and back

Day 5:

30 minutes of vigorous riding or walking
Three sets of ten to twelve side leg lifts (laying on the side).
3 sets of 10–12 push-ups (complete or on your knees)
3 sets of 10–12 repetitions using a dumbbell for single-arm rows
Stretching for ten minutes, with an emphasis on the hips, glutes, and core

Day 6:

30 minutes of tai chi or yoga
Three sets of calf lifts, 10–12 repetitions each (on a step or flat surface)
Dumbbell chest fly repetitions: three sets of ten to twelve reps
Three sets of dumbbell lateral raises (10–12 reps)
Stretching for ten minutes with an emphasis on full-body flexibility

Day 7: Rest and recovery day

Please wait, Your Review is Very Important...

Dear Reader,

I hope this message finds you well. Thank you for choosing to read the Noom Cookbook For Beginners. Your feedback is incredibly valuable to me, and I would love to hear your thoughts on the book. Whether you've just started, are halfway through, or have finished reading, your perspective matters.

Your feedback is immensely appreciated and will help me enhance future works.

Thank you for taking the time to share your thoughts on the Noom Cookbook For Beginners. Your support means the world to me.

Happy reading!

Dr. Valerie Kennedy

Chapter 8: Measurements and Conversions

The goal of carb cycling is to maximize your metabolism and encourage fat loss by rotating between days with high, moderate, and low carbohydrate intake. You'll need to know how to measure and convert your carbs in order to use carb cycling efficiently.

1. Establish your daily calorie requirements:

Use this algorithm to determine your Basal Metabolic Rate (BMR):

BMR = 655 + (9.6 x weight in kg) + (1.7 x height in cm) - (4.7 x age)

Depending on how active you are, multiply your BMR by an activity factor.

- Sedentary (little to no exercise): BMR x 1.2
- Light activity (1-3 days per week): BMR x 1.375
- Moderate activity (3-5 days per week): BMR x 1.55
- Very active (6-7 days per week): BMR x 1.725
- Extra active (very active + physical job): BMR x 1.9
- The result is your estimated daily caloric needs.

2. Set your daily carb intake:

High-carb day: 50% of your daily caloric intake should come from carbs

Moderate-carb day: 30% of your daily caloric intake should come from carbs

Low-carb day: 20% of your daily caloric intake should come from carbs

3. Convert grams of carbs to calories:

1 gram of carbohydrate contains 4 calories

Example: If your daily caloric needs are 2000 calories and you want to consume 50% of your calories from carbs on a high-carb day:

50% of 2000 calories = 1000 calories from carbs

1000 calories / 4 calories per gram = 250 grams of carbs

4. Convert grams of carbs to ounces:

1 ounce (oz) of a carbohydrate-rich food typically contains 28 grams of carbs

Example: If you want to consume 250 grams of carbs on a high-carb day:

250 grams / 28 grams per oz = 8.93 oz of carbohydrate-rich food

5. Meal planning tips for carb cycling:

High-carb day: Focus on whole grains, fruits, and starchy vegetables
Moderate-carb day: Include a mix of whole grains, fruits, and non-starchy vegetables
Low-carb day: Emphasize non-starchy vegetables and lean protein sources

Bonus: Video Course

Click or type in the link on your browser or you can scan the QR code for each of the videos.

Module 1: Carb Cycling Basics

http://tinyurl.com/7urfjpnc

Module 2: Meal Planning and Preparation

http://tinyurl.com/38ubzjwf

Module 3: Exercise and Fitness

http://tinyurl.com/38vf5hay

Module 4: Staying Motivated and Overcoming Challenges

http://tinyurl.com/ytmkvdh4

Conclusion

A versatile and successful weight reduction strategy is carb cycling, particularly for women over 50 who want to increase their energy, gain strength, and reduce weight. You may improve your metabolism and reach your weight reduction goals while still indulging in your favorite meals by switching up your diet with high-carb and low-carb days.

We have given you a thorough introduction to carb cycling in this book, along with simple-to-follow workout routines, mouthwatering meals, and a 21-day eating plan. The extra audiobook and video course provide further help and direction, making sure you have all you need to be successful.

You will gain strength and increase your energy by using the workout routines and recipes in this book together with the carb cycling concepts. You will also lose weight. This will enable you to maintain an active and satisfying lifestyle as you age.

Keep in mind that benefits from your carb cycling adventure may not come right away, so be patient and persistent. To make sure your carb cycling program is effective for you, pay attention to your body and modify it as necessary.

I hope this book has given you the information and resources you need to confidently start your carb cycling adventure. I'm wishing you well and eager to hear about your accomplishments in terms of energy, strength, and weight reduction.

Please wait, Your Review is Very Important…

Dear Reader,

I hope this message finds you well. Thank you for choosing to read the Noom Cookbook For Beginners. Your feedback is incredibly valuable to me, and I would love to hear your thoughts

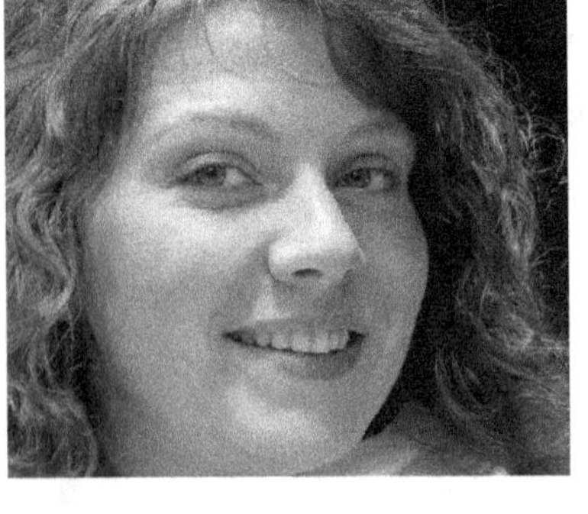

on the book. Whether you've just started, are halfway through, or have finished reading, your perspective matters.

Your feedback is immensely appreciated and will help me enhance future works.

Thank you for taking the time to share your thoughts on the Noom Cookbook For Beginners. Your support means the world to me.

Happy reading!

Dr. Valerie Kennedy

www.ingramcontent.com/pod-product-compliance
Lightning Source LLC
Chambersburg PA
CBHW081436250726
48662CB00009B/2812